T0259552

# Aspirin-Exacerbated Respiratory Disease

*Editor*

ANDREW A. WHITE

# IMMUNOLOGY AND ALLERGY CLINICS OF NORTH AMERICA

www.immunology.theclinics.com

*Consulting Editor*
STEPHEN A. TILLES

November 2016 • Volume 36 • Number 4

**ELSEVIER**

1600 John F. Kennedy Boulevard • Suite 1800 • Philadelphia, Pennsylvania, 19103-2899
http://www.theclinics.com

**IMMUNOLOGY AND ALLERGY CLINICS OF NORTH AMERICA Volume 36, Number 4**
**November 2016 ISSN 0889-8561, ISBN-13: 978-0-323-47685-0**

Editor: Jessica McCool
Developmental Editor: Kristen Helm

© **2016 Elsevier Inc. All rights reserved.**

This periodical and the individual contributions contained in it are protected under copyright by Elsevier, and the following terms and conditions apply to their use:

**Photocopying**

Single photocopies of single articles may be made for personal use as allowed by national copyright laws. Permission of the Publisher and payment of a fee is required for all other photocopying, including multiple or systematic copying, copying for advertising or promotional purposes, resale, and all forms of document delivery. Special rates are available for educational institutions that wish to make photocopies for non-profit educational classroom use. For information on how to seek permission visit www.elsevier.com/permissions or call: (+44) 1865 843830 (UK)/(+1) 215 239 3804 (USA).

**Derivative Works**

Subscribers may reproduce tables of contents or prepare lists of articles including abstracts for internal circulation within their institutions. Permission of the Publisher is required for resale or distribution outside the institution. Permission of the Publisher is required for all other derivative works, including compilations and translations (please consult www.elsevier.com/permissions).

**Electronic Storage or Usage**

Permission of the Publisher is required to store or use electronically any material contained in this periodical, including any article or part of an article (please consult www.elsevier.com/permissions). Except as outlined above, no part of this publication may be reproduced, stored in a retrieval system or transmitted in any form or by any means, electronic, mechanical, photocopying, recording or otherwise, without prior written permission of the Publisher.

**Notice**

No responsibility is assumed by the Publisher for any injury and/or damage to persons or property as a matter of products liability, negligence or otherwise, or from any use or operation of any methods, products, instructions or ideas contained in the material herein. Because of rapid advances in the medical sciences, in particular, independent verification of diagnoses and drug dosages should be made.

Although all advertising material is expected to conform to ethical (medical) standards, inclusion in this publication does not constitute a guarantee or endorsement of the quality or value of such product or of the claims made of it by its manufacturer.

*Immunology and Allergy Clinics of North America* (ISSN 0889–8561) is published quarterly by Elsevier Inc., 360 Park Avenue South, New York, NY 10010-1710. Months of issue are February, May, August, and November. Periodicals postage paid at New York, NY and additional mailing offices. Subscription prices are $320.00 per year for US individuals, $508.00 per year for US institutions, $100.00 per year for US students and residents, $395.00 per year for Canadian individuals, $220.00 per year for Canadian students, $644.00 per year for Canadian institutions, $445.00 per year for international individuals, $644.00 per year for international institutions, $220.00 per year for international students. To receive student/resident rate, orders must be accompanied by name of affiliated institution, date of term, and the *signature* of program/residency coordinator on institution letterhead. Orders will be billed at individual rate until proof of status is received. Foreign air speed delivery is included in all *Clinics* subscription prices. All prices are subject to change without notice. **POSTMASTER**: Send address changes to *Immunology and Allergy Clinics of North America,* Elsevier Health Sciences Division, Subscription Customer Service, 3251 Riverport Lane, Maryland Heights, MO 63043. **Customer Service: 1-800-654-2452 (U.S. and Canada); 314-447-8871 (outside U.S. and Canada). Fax: 314-447-8029. E-mail: journalscustomerservice-usa@elsevier.com (for print support); journalsonlinesupport-usa@elsevier.com (for online support).**

*Reprints.* For copies of 100 or more, of articles in this publication, please contact the Commercial Reprints Department, Elsevier Inc., 360 Park Avenue South, New York, New York 10010-1710. Tel. 212-633-3874, Fax: 212-633-3820, E-mail: reprints@elsevier.com.

*Immunology and Allergy Clinics of North America is covered in MEDLINE/PubMed (Index Medicus), Current Contents/Life Sciences, Science Citation Index, ISI/BIOMED, Chemical Abstracts, and EMBASE/Excerpta Medica.*

# Contributors

## CONSULTING EDITOR

**STEPHEN A. TILLES, MD**
Executive Director, ASTHMA Inc Clinical Research Center; Partner, Northwest Asthma and Allergy Center; Clinical Professor of Medicine, University of Washington, Seattle, Washington

## EDITOR

**ANDREW A. WHITE, MD**
Director, AERD Program, Division of Allergy, Asthma and Immunology, Scripps Clinic, San Diego, California

## AUTHORS

**MATTHEW C. ALTMAN, MD**
Assistant Professor, Allergy Section, Division of Allergy and Infectious Diseases, Department of Medicine, UW Medicine, University of Washington, Seattle, Washington

**ANDREW G. AYARS, MD**
Assistant Professor, Allergy Section, Division of Allergy and Infectious Diseases, Department of Medicine, UW Medicine, University of Washington, Seattle, Washington

**LARRY BORISH, MD**
Professor, Departments of Medicine and Microbiology, Asthma and Allergic Disease Center, Carter Center for Immunology Research, University of Virginia Health System, Charlottesville, Virginia

**TREVER BURNETT, MD**
Physician, Northwest Asthma and Allergy Center, Seattle, Washington

**KATHERINE N. CAHILL, MD**
Instructor, Division of Rheumatology, Immunology and Allergy, Brigham and Women's Hospital, Harvard Medical School, Boston, Massachusetts

**AMBER DAHLIN, PhD, MMSc**
Channing Division of Network Medicine, Brigham and Women's Hospital, Harvard Medical School, Boston, Massachusetts

**WILLIAM R. HENDERSON Jr, MD**
Professor, Allergy Section, Division of Allergy and Infectious Diseases, Department of Medicine, UW Medicine, University of Washington, Seattle, Washington

**JENNIFER HILL, MD**
Fellow, Adult Program, Division of Allergy and Immunology, National Jewish Health, University of Colorado, Denver, Colorado

**ROHIT KATIAL, MD, FAAAAI, FACP**
Professor of Medicine; Associate Vice President of Clinical Research; Helen Wohlberg & Herman Lambert Chair in Pharmacokinetics, Division of Allergy and Immunology; Co-Director of the Cohen Asthma Institute, National Jewish Health, University of Colorado, Denver, Colorado

**MAREK L. KOWALSKI, MD, PhD**
Department of Immunology, Rheumatology and Allergy, Healthy Ageing Research Center, Medical University of Łódź, Łódź, Poland

**TANYA M. LAIDLAW, MD**
Assistant Professor, Division of Rheumatology, Immunology and Allergy, Brigham and Women's Hospital, Harvard Medical School, Boston, Massachusetts

**JOANNA S. MAKOWSKA, MD, PhD**
Department of Rheumatology, Medical University of Łódź, Łódź, Poland

**ANDREW R. PARKER, MD**
Senior Fellow, Allergy Section, Division of Allergy and Infectious Diseases, Department of Medicine, UW Medicine, University of Washington, Seattle, Washington

**SPENCER C. PAYNE, MD**
Associate Professor, Departments of Medicine and Otolaryngology – Head and Neck Surgery, University of Virginia Health System, Charlottesville, Virginia

**ROBERT P. SCHLEIMER, PhD**
The Roy and Elaine Patterson Professor, Division of Allergy-Immunology, Department of Medicine; Department of Otolaryngology, Northwestern University Feinberg School of Medicine, Chicago, Illinois

**RONALD A. SIMON, MD**
Head, Department of Allergy and Immunology, Scripps Clinic Carmel Valley, Scripps Clinic, San Diego, California

**JOHN W. STEINKE, PhD**
Associate Professor, Department of Medicine, Asthma and Allergic Disease Center, Carter Center for Immunology Research, University of Virginia Health System, Charlottesville, Virginia

**WHITNEY W. STEVENS, MD, PhD**
Instructor, Division of Allergy-Immunology, Department of Medicine, Northwestern University Feinberg School of Medicine, Chicago, Illinois

**DONALD D. STEVENSON, MD**
Division of Allergy, Asthma and Immunology, Scripps Clinic, San Diego, California

**JEREMY D. WALDRAM, MD**
Department of Allergy and Immunology, Scripps Clinic Carmel Valley, Scripps Clinic, San Diego, California

**KRISTEN M. WALTERS, MD**
Department of Allergy, Asthma & Immunology, Scripps Clinic, San Diego, California

**ALEKSANDRA WARDZYŃSKA, MD, PhD**
Department of Immunology, Rheumatology and Allergy, Healthy Ageing Research Center, Medical University of Łódź, Łódź, Poland

**SCOTT T. WEISS, MD, MS**
Channing Division of Network Medicine, Brigham and Women's Hospital, Harvard Medical School, Boston, Massachusetts

**ANDREW A. WHITE, MD**
Director, AERD Program, Division of Allergy, Asthma and Immunology, Scripps Clinic, San Diego, California

**ADAM N. WILLIAMS, MD**
Chair, Department of Allergy, Asthma, and Immunology, Bend Memorial Clinic, Bend, Oregon; Affiliate Clinical Professor, School of Medicine, Oregon Health and Sciences University, Portland, Oregon

**KATHARINE M. WOESSNER, MD**
Program Director, Allergy and Immunology Fellowship Program, Department of Allergy, Asthma & Immunology, Scripps Clinic, San Diego, California

# Contents

> Nonsteroidal antiinflammatory drugs (NSAIDs), including aspirin, are among the most commonly used drugs worldwide. They account for a large number of adverse drug reactions (ADRs). The prevalence of NSAID-induced reactions is increasing. Distinguishing between a predicted side effect of a drug and a potentially life-threatening hypersensitivity reaction is essential to manage the affected patient. However, most clinicians find it difficult to diagnose these types of reactions despite published classification schemes. In this overview, we provide an in-depth review of NSAID classification, types of NSAID reactions, diagnostic tactics, and management strategies to provide the reader with a greater understanding of NSAID-induced reactions.

> Aspirin-exacerbated respiratory disease is a significant endotype of both asthma and chronic rhinosinusitis with nasal polyps. The disease demonstrates what seems to be a unified inflammatory mechanism culminating in highly eosinophilic nasal polyp disease and asthma. The rate of polyp recurrence and morbidity from asthma exacerbations are significant and warrant separating this group diagnostically from aspirin-tolerant peers. Given the unique anti-inflammatory effects of aspirin and the evolving landscape of new, targeted biologic treatments, it is even more incumbent to consider this diagnosis and offer patients treatment specific for the disease.

> Aspirin-exacerbated respiratory disease (AERD) is a distinct clinical condition characterized by chronic sinusitis with nasal polyps, asthma, and hypersensitivity reactions to nonsteroidal anti-inflammatory drugs (NSAIDs). Distinguishing AERD from other forms of chronic sinusitis, asthma, and

NSAID reactivity has important clinical implications for management. The clinical history is helpful, but not adequate for confirming the diagnosis of AERD, in most cases. Diagnostic provocation challenge remains the only way to confirm or exclude the diagnosis of AERD. This article discusses the utility of the clinical history and the current evidence regarding measures that optimize the safety of performing diagnostic NSAID provocation challenges.

Aspirin-exacerbated respiratory disease (AERD) and Chronic Rhinosinusitis with Nasal Polyps (CRSwNP) are both characterized by the presence of chronic sinonasal inflammation and nasal polyps. Unlike in CRSwNP, AERD patients develop respiratory reactions following ingestion of COX-1 inhibitors. AERD patients also, on average, have worse upper respiratory disease with increased sinonasal symptoms, mucosal inflammation and requirements for revision sinus surgery when compared to CRSwNP patients. While no single genetic factor has been identified in either CRSwNP or AERD to date, differences in the metabolism of arachidonic acid as well as innate immune cell activation may uniquely contribute to AERD pathogenesis.

The acute clinical symptoms that develop following the oral ingestion of aspirin, or any other inhibitor of cyclooxygenase-1, are well established in aspirin-exacerbated respiratory disease: nasal congestion, rhinorrhea, and bronchospasm. Less commonly, gastrointestinal distress, rash, angioedema, or urticaria also develops. However, the pathobiology that drives these clinical reactions is poorly understood. Use of an intranasal aspirin challenge protocol or administration of premedications inhibiting the leukotriene pathway decreases the severity of clinical reaction, which suggests the involvement of both local effector cells and cysteinyl leukotrienes in the pathogenesis of aspirin-induced reactions.

Aspirin-exacerbated respiratory disease (AERD) is characterized by chronic rhinosinusitis with nasal polyps, asthma, and reactions to cyclooxygenase-1–inhibiting drugs. This condition is often refractory to standard medical treatments and results in aggressive nasal polyposis that often requires multiple sinus surgeries. Aspirin desensitization followed by daily aspirin therapy is an important treatment option, and its efficacy has been validated in multiple research studies. Aspirin desensitization is not without risk, but specific protocols and recommendations exist to mitigate the risk. Most patients with AERD can undergo aspirin desensitization in an outpatient setting under the supervision of an allergist.

The clinical efficacy of aspirin treatment after desensitization in patients with respiratory disease exacerbated by nonsteroidal anti-inflammatory drugs has been documented in observational studies and in double-blind placebo-controlled trials. There is no general agreement with regard to the optimal maintenance dose or duration of treatment with acetylsalicylic acid after desensitization, thus further studies are necessary to offer clear guidelines to clinicians. This article summarizes data from noncontrolled, active-control, and placebo-controlled trials assessing clinical effectiveness and reporting on safety of treatment with acetylsalicylic acid in desensitized patients with respiratory disease exacerbated by nonsteroidal anti-inflammatory drugs.

Aspirin-exacerbated respiratory disease (AERD) involves overexpression of proinflammatory mediators, including 5-lipoxygenase and leukotriene $C_4$ synthase ($LTC_4S$), resulting in constitutive overproduction of cysteinyl leukotrienes. Mast cells and eosinophils have roles in mediating many of the observed effects. Increased levels of both interleukin-4 (IL-4) and interferon (IFN)-$\gamma$ are present in the tissue of patients with AERD. Previous studies showed that IL-4 is primarily responsible for the upregulation of $LTC_4S$ by mast cells. Our studies show that IFN-$\gamma$, but not IL-4, drives this process in eosinophils. This article examines the overall role that eosinophils and mast cells contribute to the pathophysiology of AERD.

Aspirin-exacerbated respiratory disease (AERD) is a clinical syndrome characterized by severe persistent asthma, hyperplastic eosinophilic sinusitis with nasal polyps, and an intolerance to aspirin and other NSAIDs that preferentially inhibit COX-1. For more than 30 years, aspirin desensitization has proven to be of significant long-term benefit in carefully selected patients with AERD. Despite this, the exact mechanisms behind the therapeutic effects of aspirin desensitization remain poorly understood. In this article, we review the current understanding of the mechanisms of aspirin desensitization and discuss future areas of investigation.

Aspirin-exacerbated respiratory disease (AERD) is a syndrome of severe asthma and rhinosinusitis with nasal polyposis with exacerbations of baseline eosinophil-driven and mast cell–driven inflammation after nonsteroidal antiinflammatory drug ingestion. Although the underlying pathophysiology is poorly understood, dysregulation of the cyclooxygenase and 5-lipoxygenase pathways of arachidonic acid metabolism is thought to be key. Central features of AERD pathogenesis are overproduction of proinflammatory and bronchoconstrictor cysteinyl leukotrienes and prostaglandin (PG) $D_2$ and inhibition of bronchoprotective and antiinflammatory $PGE_2$. Imbalance in the ratio of these lipid mediators likely leads to the increased eosinophilic and mast cell inflammatory responses in the respiratory tract.

Amber Dahlin and Scott T. Weiss

Aspirin-exacerbated respiratory disease (AERD) severity and its clinical phenotypes are characterized by genetic variation within pathways for arachidonic acid metabolism, inflammation, and immune responses. Epigenetic effects, including DNA methylation and histone protein modification, contribute to regulation of many genes that contribute to inflammatory states in AERD. The development of noninvasive, predictive clinical tests using data from genetic, epigenetic, pharmacogenetic, and biomarker studies will improve precision medicine efforts for AERD and asthma treatment.

# IMMUNOLOGY AND ALLERGY CLINICS OF NORTH AMERICA

**THE CLINICS ARE AVAILABLE ONLINE!**
Access your subscription at:
www.theclinics.com

# IMMUNOLOGY AND ALLERGY
# CLINICS OF NORTH AMERICA

## FORTHCOMING ISSUES

**February 2017**
Allergic Skin Diseases
Peter S. Lio, and
Peter Schmid-Grendelmeier, Editors

**May 2017**
Biologic Therapy of Immunologic Diseases
Bradley E. Chipps and Stephen P. Peters,
Editors

**August 2017**
Angioedema
Marc Riedl, Editor

## RECENT ISSUES

**August 2016**
Severe Asthma
Rohit K. Katial, Editor

**May 2016**
Rhinitis
Jonathan A. Bernstein, Editor

**February 2016**
Aeroallergen and Food Immunotherapy
Linda S. Cox and
Anna H. Nowak-Wegrzyn, Editors

## ISSUE OF RELATED INTEREST

Emergency Medicine Clinics of North America, February 2016 (Vol. 34, No. 1)
Respiratory Emergencies
Robert J. Vissers and Michael A. Gibbs, Editors
Available at: http://www.emed.theclinics.com

**THE CLINICS ARE AVAILABLE ONLINE!**
Access your subscription at:
www.theclinics.com

# Foreword

# From "Samter's Triad" to "NERD": The Long and Winding Road to Understanding Aspirin-Exacerbated Respiratory Disease

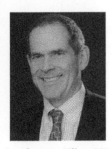

Stephen A. Tilles, MD
*Consulting Editor*

Depending on where you trained, you may have learned about "Samter's triad," "triad asthma," "ASA-induced asthma with nasal polyposis," "aspirin-exacerbated respiratory disease" (AERD), or even "NSAID-Exacerbated Respiratory Disease." Each of these names represents an attempt to categorize the same group of our most challenging patients, and this well-meaning but confusing nomenclature reflects the inherent difficulty encountered when trying to bridge the gap between clinical descriptions and a true understanding of this unique syndrome. We have known for decades that patients with this condition are no more likely to be atopic than the general population, suggesting early on that pathways to eosinophilic inflammation exist that are not dependent on IgE recognition of an allergen. Fortunately, in recent years there has been significant progress made in describing the pathophysiology of AERD. This issue of *Immunology and Allergy Clinics of North America* provides detailed reviews of our current understanding of the AERD endotype, including the roles of mast cells, eosinophils, and lipid mediators, as well as an updated description of how cyclo-oxygenase inhibition results in such an explosive onset of clinical symptoms. In addition, there are three separate articles on aspirin therapy. The first article summarizes its mechanisms; the second reviews clinical trial data, and the third details safe and effective approaches to achieve clinical benefit.

The group of authors assembled by guest editor, Andrew White, for this issue of *Immunology and Allergy Clinics of North America* includes both "giants" in the field

Immunol Allergy Clin N Am 36 (2016) xiii–xiv
http://dx.doi.org/10.1016/j.iac.2016.08.002
0889-8561/16/© 2016 Published by Elsevier Inc.

**immunology.theclinics.com**

who have conducted active investigation and systematic clinical AERD care their entire careers as well as early and mid-career AERD experts who provide complementary insights. I think you will agree that this collection of articles will serve as an essential reference for both trainees and practicing specialists who take care of AERD patients, including Allergy/Asthma specialists, Pulmonologists, and Otolaryngologists.

Stephen A. Tilles, MD
ASTHMA Inc Clinical Research Center
Northwest Asthma and Allergy Center
University of Washington
9725 Third Avenue, NE, Suite 500
Seattle, WA 98115, USA

E-mail address:
stilles@nwasthma.com

# Preface

# Aspirin-Exacerbated Respiratory Disease: The Hunt for the "Rosetta Stone" of Respiratory Inflammation

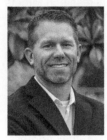

Andrew A. White, MD
*Editor*

Undecipherable for centuries, Egyptian hieroglyphics persistently resisted attempts at translation. Since they were unable to interpret this written language form, archeologists and explorers stared in wonder, albeit perplexedly, at the written history of the Pharaohs, Queens, and Priests inscribed on the walls around them. This left the 3000-year history of the ancient Egyptians lost to modern understanding. Deciphering the hieroglyphics might never have occurred were it not for the discovery of the Rosetta Stone in 1799, an ancient stone inscribed with a royal decree in three written forms: Greek, Demotic script, and ancient Egyptian hieroglyphics. With the discovery of the Rosetta Stone, the key to the discovery of hieroglyph translation materialized. Greek scholars were able to slowly piece together the meaning of some scattered hieroglyphic symbols. Although the three scripts were communicating the same message, it was only by consolidating the work of multiple researchers in the subsequent 20 years that Champollion was able to generate a thorough list of Egyptian symbols in 1821 and crack the code. This ushered in a renaissance in the study of ancient Egyptian culture.

A similar occurrence is crucial in the investigation of aspirin-exacerbated respiratory disease (AERD). Since its first description in 1922, nearly 100 years later, we still do not have an explanation for the relatively sudden development of the disease in healthy individuals. As a specific endotype of asthma and chronic rhinosinusitis with nasal polyposis, unraveling the mechanisms in AERD could dramatically illumine our understanding of type 2 airway inflammation. Although chronic rhinosinusitis and asthma are multifactorial in their genesis, the stereotypical onset of AERD begs for a singular explanation. Were we able to define the event that "turns on" AERD, it would

Immunol Allergy Clin N Am 36 (2016) xv–xvi
http://dx.doi.org/10.1016/j.iac.2016.08.001
0889-8561/16/© 2016 Published by Elsevier Inc.

immunology.theclinics.com

truly be a watershed moment in understanding environmentally triggered chronic eosinophilic respiratory disease. The last five years have produced many successful research endeavors that have whittled away at the enigma of AERD. However, we still do not see things clearly. Several basic mechanistic questions evade explanation. Similar to adventurers with a golden sarcophagus before them, yet unable to even name the individual it contained until the language could be properly translated, we understand that AERD holds tremendous clues to type 2 respiratory inflammation. We just don't yet know what those are.

These articles outline the advances in the various facets of this perplexing disease, on both a basic science and clinical level. The authors connect new research findings to our expanding disease paradigm. They point toward translational research targets designed to understand mechanisms and then take these answers to the patient in the form of a targeted treatment.

Andrew A. White, MD
Division of Allergy, Asthma, and Immunology
Scripps Clinic
3811 Valley Centre Drive, S99
San Diego, CA 92130, USA

E-mail address:
white.andrew@scrippshealth.org

# An Overview of Nonsteroidal Antiinflammatory Drug Reactions

Kristen M. Walters, MD, Katharine M. Woessner, MD*

## KEYWORDS

- Nonsteroidal antiinflammatory drugs (NSAIDs) • NSAID-induced asthma
- NSAID-induced urticaria • NSAID reactions • NSAID hypersensitivity
- Aspirin intolerance • Drug allergy

## KEY POINTS

- Adverse reactions owing to ingestion of nonsteroidal antiinflammatory drugs (NSAIDs) can manifest as an array of symptoms, from mild gastrointestinal upset up to life-threatening anaphylaxis.
- NSAID-induced hypersensitivity may be divided into immunologic and nonimmunologic reactions and should be differentiated from the predictable side effects of the drug.
- The pathophysiology underlying hypersensitivity reactions is related to cyclooxygenase-1 inhibition (nonimmunologic type) or typical IgE-mediated reactions (immunologic type).
- Although difficult, it is imperative to appropriately diagnosis and categorize the type of NSAID-induced reaction so that the affected patient may be managed effectively.

## INTRODUCTION

Since the introduction of the first nonsteroidal antiinflammatory drug (NSAID) to medical practice in the late 1800s, NSAIDs, including aspirin (ASA), have become one of the most commonly used class of drugs in the world. It is estimated that more than 20 million people in the United States use an NSAID on a consistent basis,[1] and this number is steadily increasing owing to our aging population and subsequent treatment of various inflammatory and cardiovascular conditions. Consequently, the number of adverse reactions owing to NSAID ingestion have paralleled the increase in NSAID use and may account for up to 10% of preventable drug-related hospital admissions.[2] These reactions vary in severity, from mild gastrointestinal (GI) or cutaneous symptoms, to severe life-threatening anaphylaxis.

---

Disclosure Statement: The authors have nothing to disclose.
Department of Allergy, Asthma & Immunology, Scripps Clinic, 3811 Valley Centre Drive, San Diego, CA 92130, USA
* Corresponding author.
*E-mail address:* Woessner.katharine@scrippshealth.org

Immunol Allergy Clin N Am 36 (2016) 625–641
http://dx.doi.org/10.1016/j.iac.2016.06.001
0889-8561/16/$ – see front matter © 2016 Elsevier Inc. All rights reserved.

The ability to distinguish between a suspected, but unwanted, side effect of a medication and a true hypersensitivity reaction is paramount but frequently met with challenge. In addition to the wide range of symptoms that characterize these reactions, they are often accompanied by abnormal immunologic and/or nonimmunologic processes, which can further complicate the clinician's ability to diagnose and manage NSAID-induced reactions.

Over the years, several classification schemes have been proposed to assist the clinician in identifying and understanding the different forms of NSAID hypersensitivity reactions. In this review, these classification strategies will be used to provide the reader with an in-depth overview of the clinical presentation and management of both immunologic and nonimmunologic NSAID reactions.

## MECHANISM AND CLASSIFICATION OF NONSTEROIDAL ANTI-INFLAMMATORY DRUGS

It is well-understood that NSAIDs, including ASA, share a common pharmacologic method of action via the inhibition of cyclooxygenase (COX) enzymes. The inhibition of COX leads to altered arachidonic acid metabolism and decreased formation of prostaglandins, prostacyclin, and thromboxanes (**Fig. 1**).[3] Two isoforms of COX have been described, COX-1 and COX-2:

- *COX-1*: Often referred to as the "housekeeping" enzyme owing to its role in maintaining various protective cellular functions, such as the integrity of gastric mucosa, platelet aggregation, and renal function, via production of prostanoids.[4] It is constitutively expressed by most human cell types.
- *COX-2*: Expression is primarily induced in response to inflammatory or mitogenic stimuli (eg, interleukin-1, endotoxin), and inhibited by glucocorticoids. It is constitutively expressed in specific cell types with physiologic roles in reproduction, bone reabsorption, renal function, and neurotransmission.[5] There exists a potential association between COX-2 and adverse cardiovascular outcomes, but this remains to be fully elucidated.[6,7]

The strength of enzyme inhibition is known to vary among the different NSAIDs and explains their ability to generate different levels of clinical effectiveness, side effects, and hypersensitivity reactions.

In general, NSAIDs that inhibit COX-1 are considered to be "cross-reactive" with ASA (eg, ibuprofen, naproxen, ketorolac). NSAIDs that inhibit both COX isoforms are considered "nonselective." Highly selective COX-2 inhibitors have a 200- to 300-fold selectivity for COX-2 at approved therapeutic doses. The 4 broad categories of COX inhibition are listed as follows (**Box 1**):

- Highly selective COX-1 inhibitors
- Weakly selective COX-1 inhibitors
- Preferentially selective COX-2 inhibitors
- Highly selective COX-2 inhibitors

Despite all NSAIDs sharing a similar mechanism of action, it is important to note that they demonstrate differences in their chemical structure (**Table 1**). This enables certain NSAIDs to have antigenic activity and elicit a drug-specific immunologic response. It is vital that the clinician has a sound understanding of the pharmacologic properties of NSAIDs, including their mechanisms of action and degree of COX-1/COX-2 selectivity and chemical structure, to appropriately diagnose and efficiently manage any NSAID-induced reaction.

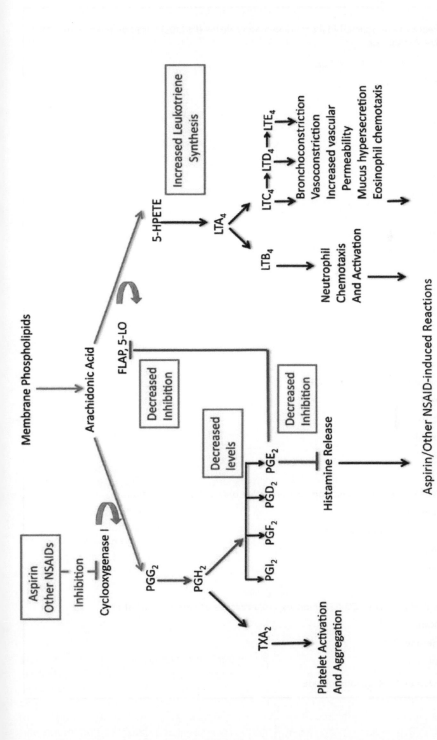

**Fig. 1.** Alteration of arachidonic acid metabolism in nonsteroidal antiinflammatory drugs (NSAID)-induced reactions after inhibition of cyclooxygenase I (COX-I). 5-HPETE, 5-hydroperoxyeicosatetraenoic acid; 5-LO, 5-lipoxygenase; FLAP, 5-lipoxygenase-activating protein; LT, leukotriene; PG, prostaglandin; TX, thromboxane. (*Adapted from* Woessner KM, Simon RA. Cardiovascular prophylaxis and aspirin "allergy". Immunol Allergy Clin North Am 2013;33(2):264; with permission.)

**Box 1**
**Cross-reactivity of nonsteroidal antiinflammatory drugs (NSAIDs) based on potency of COX-1 and COX-2 inhibition**

*Highly selective COX-1 inhibitors*

Acetylsalicylic acid

Diclofenac

Etodolac

Fenoprofen

Ibuprofen

Indomethacin

Ketoprofen

Ketorolac

Naproxen

Naproxen sodium

Mefanamic acid

Oxaprozin

Piroxicam

Sulindac

Tolmetin

*Highly selective COX-2 inhibitors*

Celecoxib

Etoricoxib

Lumiracoxib

Parecoxib

*Weakly selective COX-1 inhibitors; cross-reactive only at high concentrations*

Acetaminophen

Choline magnesium trisalicylate

Diflunisal

Salsalate

*Preferentially selective COX-2 inhibitors; cross-reactive at high concentrations*

Meloxicam

Nabumetone

Nimesulide

*Abbreviation:* COX, cyclooxygenase.

**Table 1**
Examples of NSAIDs based on chemical structure

| Salicylic Acid Derivatives | | Para-Aminophenol Derivative | Phenyl-Propionic Acids | Pyrano-Indoleacetic Acids (Acetic Acids) | Enolic Acid Derivatives (Oxicams) | Anthranilic Acids (Fenamates) |
|---|---|---|---|---|---|---|
| Acetylated | Nonacetylated | Acetaminophen (paracetamol [APAP]) | Fenoprofen | Diclofenac | Meloxicam | Meclofenamic acid (meclofenamate) |
| Acetylsalicyclic acid (aspirin [ASA]) | Choline | | Flurbiprofen | Etodolac | Piroxicam | Mefenamic acid |
| | Magnesium | | Ibuprofen | Indomethacin | Tenoxicam | |
| | Trisalicylate | | Ketoprofen | Sulindac | | |
| | Diflunisal | | Naproxen | Tolmetin | | |
| | Salsalate | | Oxaprozin | | | |
| | Sodium salicylate | | | | | |

*Abbreviation:* NSAIDs, nonsteroidal antiinflammatory drugs.

## CLASSIFICATION OF ADVERSE DRUG REACTIONS

An ADR describes any unpleasant and/or unwanted reaction that results from ingestion of a particular medication. ADRs are divided into 2 categories, types A and B:

- *Type A*: Make up the majority of ADRs (85%–90%). Distinguished by their predictable nature (ie, symptoms can arise in any individual and risk is increased
  with higher doses and/or repeated exposure to the drug). The reaction results
  from the known pharmacologic properties of the medication.
  *Examples:* Gastritis owing to chronic NSAID use; tinnitus from high-dose ASA
  use.

- *Type B*: Represents 10% to 15% of all ADRs. Reactions are not predictable, not
  dose dependent, and only occur in susceptible patients.
  *Examples:* NSAID-exacerbated cutaneous disease (NECD); anaphylaxis to
  ibuprofen.

Type B reactions can be further subclassified as follows:

- Exaggerated sensitivity to known drug toxicities;
- Idiosyncratic drug reactions; and
- Hypersensitivity drug reactions:
  ○ Nonimmunologic; and
  ○ Immunologic.

### Exaggerated Sensitivity to Known Drug Toxicities

This is similar to a type A reaction because it results from a known and predictable
pharmacologic property of the drug. However, the toxicity occurs after exposure to
a low and/or subtherapeutic concentration of medication, likely owing to altered
drug metabolism or increased end-organ sensitivity to the particular drug.
   Example: Onset of tinnitus after a single dose of ASA.

### Idiosyncratic Drug Reactions

These reactions are often specific to a single drug, but separate from its known pharmacologic properties. The exact mechanism remains unknown but is thought to
involve various metabolic, immune and/or genetic factors.
   Examples: Fixed drug eruptions, Stevens-Johnson syndrome, toxic epidermal necrolysis, erythema nodosum, hypersensitivity pneumonitis, aseptic meningitis, intersti-
tial nephritis, and bullous leukocytoclastic vasculitis.

### Hypersensitivity Drug Reactions

This subcategory is divided into nonimmune and immune-mediated drug reactions. The
classification of NSAID hypersensitivity reactions was originally proposed by Stevenson
and colleagues[8] to assist the clinician in identifying and understanding the specific pathophysiologic mechanisms behind each type of hypersensitivity reaction. In recent years,
a task force created by the European Academy of Allergy and Clinical Immunology presented a modified classification scheme with evidence-based recommendations for the
diagnosis and management of these reactions.[9,10] In this review, we provide a blended
classification and in-depth overview of each NSAID-induced reaction subtype.

#### Nonimmunologic hypersensitivity drug reactions

These reactions represent the majority of NSAID-induced hypersensitivity reactions.
They have been previously referred to as "pseudoallergic" reactions because they

often present with similar signs and symptoms of a typical immunologic drug reaction; however, no exact immune mechanism has been validated for these particular reactions. As such, nonimmunologic reactions are often difficult to distinguish clinically from a true allergic reaction and may create a diagnostic dilemma for the clinician.

The pathophysiology of NSAID-induced nonimmunologic reactions is not entirely known, but it is strongly tied to the inhibition of the COX-1 enzyme (see **Fig. 1**). COX-1 inhibition by either ASA or any cross-reactive NSAID results in decreased synthesis of antiinflammatory prostanoids, particularly prostaglandin $E_2$. This depletion in prostaglandin $E_2$ removes the "brake" on 5-lipoxygenase activity, thus allowing a shift toward the production of cysteinyl leukotrienes and the start of the inflammatory cascade. Decreased prostaglandin $E_2$ levels also enhance mast cell activation resulting in release of tryptase and histamine.

In general, the chance that a particular NSAID will cause a nonimmunologic reaction is highly linked to the selectivity of that NSAID for COX-1 inhibition. Given this mechanism, affected patients will almost always present with a history of reactions to several different NSAIDs, including those with dissimilar chemical structures. This is in contrast to immunologic drug reactions, in which the affected patient should only react to a single NSAID (with the exception of those that are strongly similar in chemical structure).

Nonimmunologic/nonallergic reactions can be divided into 4 subtypes (**Table 2**):

- NSAID-exacerbated asthma and rhinosinusitis;
- NSAID-exacerbated urticaria/angioedema in patients with chronic urticaria;
- NSAID-induced urticaria/angioedema (NIUA) in healthy individuals; and
- Mixed NSAID-induced reactions.

### *Asthma and rhinosinusitis exacerbated by nonsteroidal antiinflammatory drugs*

This subtype of nonimmunologic hypersensitivity reactions is characterized by onset of upper and/or lower airway symptoms upon ingestion of an NSAID in the setting of chronic rhinosinusitis, nasal polyposis, and/or asthma. This constellation of symptoms is more commonly described as "ASA-exacerbated respiratory disease" (AERD). Chronic rhinosinusitis and/or asthma often precede the onset of ASA or NSAID hypersensitivity; however, NSAID/ASA ingestion will occasionally be the precipitator of the first asthma exacerbation.

Patients typically report the onset of rhinorrhea, nasal congestion, conjunctival injection, bronchospasm, and/or laryngospasm within 30 to 180 minutes of NSAID exposure. These reactions may also be accompanied by nonrespiratory symptoms including facial flushing, urticaria, angioedema, nausea, vomiting, or diarrhea.

Clinically, these patients typically experience a more severe course of their asthma and chronic rhinosinusitis. The latter is complicated by marked eosinophilic inflammation and frequently results in recurrent nasal polyp formation requiring surgical management. NSAID-induced asthma exacerbations are a significant risk factor for fatal outcomes, and are responsible for a higher incidence of emergency room visits and hospital admissions compared with ASA-tolerant asthmatics.[11] A detailed discussion of AERD is available in later articles of this review issue.

NSAID-induced respiratory reactions are dose-dependent and related to the potency of COX-1 inhibition of the particular NSAID. As described, NSAIDs that are said to be cross-reactive with ASA are considered strong COX-1 inhibitors and subsequently have a greater risk of inducing respiratory reactions in susceptible patients. On the other hand, weak COX-1 inhibitors or selective COX-2 inhibitors are generally well-tolerated.[12]

**Table 2**
**Subtypes of nonimmunologic hypersensitivity reactions to NSAIDs**

| Reaction Subtype | Signs and Symptoms | Risk Factors |
|---|---|---|
| NSAID-induced/exacerbated asthma and rhinosinusitis | Nasoocular<br>• Rhinorrhea[a]<br>• Nasal obstruction[a]<br>• Periorbital edema<br>• Conjunctival injection[a]<br>Respiratory<br>• Throat tightness<br>• Laryngospasm<br>• Bronchospasm[a]<br>Cutaneous<br>• Skin flushing[a]<br>• Urticaria<br>Gastrointestinal<br>• Abdominal pain<br>• Nausea/vomiting | Asthma<br>Chronic rhinosinusitis<br>Nasal polyposis<br>AERD |
| NECD | Urticaria<br>Angioedema<br>Frequent involvement of the face and upper respiratory tract<br>Severity is linked to overall control of their chronic hives | Chronic urticaria (presence of hives ≥6 wk in duration)<br>Dose-dependent |
| NSAID-induced urticaria/angioedema | Urticaria<br>Angioedema<br>Isolated angioedema of the face may be seen | None, patients are generally healthy<br>Often with a history of atopic disease |
| Mixed reactions | Combination of symptoms involving the skin and respiratory tract.<br>Example: AERD patient with historical reaction to ASA (bronchospasm, nasal obstruction) who now develops cutaneous symptoms upon ASA/NSAID ingestion. | None, may be seen in healthy individuals or those with chronic disease |

*Abbreviations:* AERD, aspirin exacerbated-respiratory disease; ASA, aspirin; NECD, NSAID-exacerbated cutaneous disease; NSAIDs, nonsteroidal antiinflammatory drugs.
[a] Most commonly identified in clinical history.

## Urticaria/angioedema exacerbated by nonsteroidal antiinflammatory drugs in patients with chronic urticaria

In those patients with a history of chronic urticaria (defined by the presence of urticaria for ≥6 weeks), ingestion of COX-1 inhibiting NSAIDs can result in an acute flare of urticaria with or without concomitant angioedema. This nonimmunologic hypersensitivity reaction is known as "NSAID-exacerbated cutaneous disease." In a 2015 study, NECD was reported to affect nearly 12% of patients with underlying chronic urticaria,[13] but has been shown to be as high as 30% in other studies.[14]

Cutaneous reactions typically develop between 0.5 and 6 hours after NSAID ingestion and may last for up to 24 to 48 hours. In comparison with chronic urticaria patients without NSAID sensitivity, patients with NECD have been shown to have longer duration of their disease, a higher frequency of angioedema and atopic disease, and greater involvement of the face and upper respiratory tract.[13]

These NSAID-induced reactions are generally dose dependent and greatly influenced by the overall control of their urticaria. For example, those with active urticaria will show a greater sensitivity to cross-reactive COX-1 inhibiting NSAIDs compared with those individuals whose hives are quiescent. Thus, avoidance of these NSAIDs are helpful in reducing acute exacerbations of hives. However, it has not been shown to alter or reduce the overall disease course. For NECD patients who require antiinflammatory treatment, selective COX-2 inhibitors are generally well tolerated.[15]

### Nonsteroidal antiinflammatory drug-induced urticaria/angioedema in healthy individuals

This reaction subtype is similar to NECD; however, it is characterized by the occurrence of urticaria and/or angioedema after NSAID ingestion in asymptomatic or otherwise healthy individuals (ie, no history of chronic urticaria). These reactions typically develop within 1 to 6 hours of exposure to a COX-1 inhibiting NSAID. Isolated angioedema may be seen and is often localized to the face with particular involvement of the periorbital skin, lips, and mouth.[16]

Although affected individuals, by definition, are considered "healthy," it has been reported that up to 60% have underlying atopic disease (ie, allergic rhinitis, asthma). Sensitization to various inhalant aeroallergens and increased serum levels of total IgE are frequently identified.[17] As with other nonimmunologic reactions, the pathogenesis is thought to be tied to COX-1 inhibition. However, given the increased incidence of atopy in these patients, the involvement of IgE-related mechanisms should also be considered (but remains to be established).

Avoidance of ASA and other cross-reactive NSAIDs generally results in symptom resolution. Like patients with NECD, those affected by NIUA generally do well with selective COX-2 inhibitors. It is unknown whether individuals with NIUA are more likely to go on to develop chronic urticaria compared with the general population. However, a recent long-term study suggested no difference in overall risk between NIUA patients and healthy control subjects.[18]

### Mixed nonsteroidal antiinflammatory drug-induced reactions

Occasionally, NSAID-induced symptomatology does not fit into any of the 3 categories described and manifests as a mixed reaction of subtypes. For example, some healthy individuals (ie, without underlying AERD) can develop a combination of respiratory and cutaneous symptoms after ingestion of COX-1 inhibiting NSAIDs. Additionally, it has been reported that nearly 18% of NIUA and 10% of NECD patients develop concomitant respiratory symptoms (eg, bronchospasm) after NSAID ingestion.[19,20] The time course of symptom onset is variable, but generally similar to the other nonimmunologic hypersensitivity subtypes.

### Immunologic hypersensitivity reactions

In contrast with the nonimmunologic/pseudoallergic hypersensitivity reactions described, these reactions are thought to be allergen-induced (drug metabolite bound to a carrier protein), IgE-mediated hypersensitivity reactions. These reactions are different from the nonimmunologic subtypes in that they are provoked by a single NSAID, or occasionally by another with similar chemical structure (see **Table 1**). After exposure to the culprit NSAID, patients may experience a wide range of symptoms, from mild urticaria to life-threatening anaphylaxis, but are able to tolerate chemically dissimilar NSAIDs, including ASA.[21]

The NSAIDs most often linked with these immune responses are ibuprofen (most common in the United States), diclofenac, members of the pyrazolone class, and paracetamol.[22–24] Patients who experience these types of reactions need to have had at least one prior exposure to the particular NSAID to become sensitized to the drug. Thus, this serves as an important diagnostic clue when evaluating an individual with an NSAID-induced reaction.

Allergic hypersensitivity reactions can be divided as follows:

- Single NIUA and
- Single NSAID-induced anaphylaxis.

The difference between these 2 categories is solely based on the severity of the reaction. It is plausible that most patients with single NIUA would progress to anaphylaxis if they continued to repeatedly ingest that particular NSAID. Therefore, many experts consider these to be a single reaction and refer to it as "single NIUA/anaphylaxis."

Symptoms classically present within the first 30 to 60 minutes of NSAID ingestion, although they may arise within a matter of minutes, depending on the route of administration of the drug (ie, parental vs oral).[25] Most affected individuals are healthy (without underlying disease) and report onset of urticaria or localized angioedema after ingestion of the single NSAID. Nonetheless, up to one-third of patients may experience true anaphylaxis with risk of death.[19,23] Those patients will often have a past history of urticarial reactions to the offending NSAID, but continued to expose themselves to the drug owing to not recognizing the association of the 2 actions.

The majority of the COX-1 inhibiting NSAIDs have been implicated in reports of anaphylaxis, as well as the selective COX-2 inhibitor, celecoxib.[26,27] It is important to note that there have been no identified cases of anaphylaxis to ASA. For this reason, ASA is frequently used in oral challenge procedures during the diagnostic work-up of NSAID-induced reactions.

### Nonsteroidal antiinflammatory drug-induced delayed hypersensitivity reactions

Some experts consider this a subset of allergic hypersensitivity reactions, although the pathomechanism of these reactions are secondary to drug-specific $CD4^+$ and $CD8^+$ T lymphocyte interactions rather than an IgE-mediated process. By definition, these reactions occur more than 24 hours after drug exposure and are therefore considered a delayed type of hypersensitivity reaction. Cutaneous reactions are most commonly implicated, including maculopapular eruptions, fixed drug eruptions, and photosensitivity reactions.[28,29] Organ injury (eg, pneumonitis, nephritis) and other severe reactions (eg, Stevens-Johnson syndrome, toxic epidermal necrolysis) have also been documented.[30–32]

## DIAGNOSTIC APPROACH TO NONSTEROIDAL ANTIINFLAMMATORY DRUG-INDUCED REACTIONS

The diagnostic workup for any adverse reaction to NSAIDs is heavily weighted on obtaining a detailed history of the particular drug reaction, including the timing, symptom pattern, and intolerance to other NSAIDs, as well as the presence of medical comorbidities. At present, there are no recommended or validated skin tests or in vitro tests to confirm the diagnosis of any subtype of NSAID hypersensitivity. Referral to an allergy specialist with expertise in drug allergy is encouraged, particularly for those patients who have experienced severe reactions with NSAID ingestion and/or have a medical indication for ongoing NSAID therapy.

### History

When evaluating a patient with a history of an adverse NSAID-induced reaction, the following questions should be assessed.[33]

*Is this a predictable (type A) or unpredictable (type B/hypersensitivity) reaction?*
Type A NSAID reactions commonly manifest as GI symptoms and increased bleeding/ bruising and/or nephrotoxicity, and are strongly related to the duration and dose (higher doses = higher risk) of the drug. Type A reactions can often be prevented by reintroducing the drug at a lower dose.

*How long does it take for the reaction to develop after ingestion of a nonsteroidal antiinflammatory drug?*
NSAID hypersensitivity reactions are likely if symptoms occur within the first few hours (1–6 hours) of NSAID ingestion. However, the time to symptom onset does not determine the specific type or pathophysiology of the reaction. For example, an IgE-mediated mechanism (single NIUA/anaphylaxis ) may be considered if the reaction occurs within minutes of ingestion, but this pattern could also be seen in a nonimmune reaction (ie, NECD) if the patient is highly sensitive to the drug and is challenged with a drug dose exceeding their tolerance threshold. Reactions occurring more than 24 hours after NSAID ingestion are likely delayed-type hypersensitivity or idiosyncratic reactions.

*What are the symptoms that accompany the reaction?*
Assess for the presence of nasal (rhinorrhea, nasal congestion), ocular (periorbital edema, conjunctival injection), laryngeal (throat tightness, laryngospasm), bronchial (cough, wheezing, shortness of breath), cutaneous (urticaria, angioedema, flushing), GI (nausea, vomiting, abdominal pain, diarrhea), and cardiovascular (hypotension, chest pain) symptoms.

*Does the patient have any underlying chronic medical disease?*
In general, NSAID-exacerbated rhinosinusitis/asthma and NECD are associated with underlying disease, whereas NIUA and SINUAA commonly affect healthy individuals.

*Is there a history of intolerance to other nonsteroidal antiinflammatory drugs?*
This question is extremely important, because it allows the clinician to determine whether the patient's hypersensitivity reaction is cross-reactive to other NSAIDs (nonimmunologic) or solely connected to a single drug. A detailed history of past NSAID exposure, including name and dose of the drug, both before and after the NSAID reaction occurred should be documented. Remember that certain patients may only report sensitivity to NSAIDs of a similar chemical structure.

The clinician should also assess for the presence of ASA tolerance/intolerance. If a patient is able to tolerate ASA or other strong COX-1 inhibitors (ibuprofen, ketorolac), their previous NSAID reaction is strongly suggestive of an immunologic/allergic hypersensitivity reaction.

Some experts propose the following guidelines[34]:

- A nonimmunologic hypersensitivity reaction should be considered if there is a history of 3 or more adverse reactions to 2 or more different NSAIDs.
- An immunologic hypersensitivity reaction should be considered if there is a history of 2 or more reactions to the same NSAID with history of tolerance to another NSAID.

### Diagnostic Testing

The importance of obtaining a detailed history is not to be overlooked because there are no recommended in vitro or allergen skin tests to assist with confirming the diagnosis. Various testing modalities have been studied, including basophil activation testing, autologous serum skin testing, and analysis of genetic polymorphisms, but these have shown mixed results and therefore have not been validated for use in the diagnostic workup of ASA/NSAID hypersensitivity.[35] There have been a few cases showing a potential benefit of intradermal skin testing in the setting of single NIUA/anaphylaxis, but it has been rejected as a diagnostic tool owing to poor sensitivity and risk of systemic reactions.[10,24,36]

### Drug Challenge

Despite its diagnostic importance during evaluation of a suspected NSAID hypersensitivity reaction, a patient's clinical history has been shown to have an overall low specificity.[37] One study reported that more than 78% of patients with a past adverse reaction to an NSAID ultimately tolerated a subsequent oral challenge to that NSAID.[38] Thus, even with a supportive history, an oral drug challenge may be necessary to definitively rule in or out a diagnosis of NSAID hypersensitivity.

The strongest indication to perform a provocative oral challenge is for an affected individual who has a medical indication that warrants ongoing NSAID therapy, such as concomitant cardiovascular disease or a chronic inflammatory condition (ie, arthritis). An oral challenge enables the clinician to determine which type of reaction was present and what other NSAIDs the patient may safely tolerate in the future. With regard to patients with AERD, a positive ASA challenges confirms sensitivity to ASA and whether the patient may benefit from ASA desensitization and continuous ASA therapy.

Drug challenges are not without risk and should always be pursued with caution. Therefore, they are seldom recommended for patients with a history of an anaphylactic reaction to NSAIDs. In these situations, it is best to strictly avoid the culprit drug. General avoidance of NSAIDs is also a conservative and practical option for those patients who do not have a medical need for NSAID therapy.

Challenge protocols consist of a gradual administration of an increasing dose of NSAID (**Table 3**).[39] ASA is most often used and considered the "gold standard" of NSAID challenges because there have been no confirmed cases of anaphylaxis to the drug.

- A positive ASA challenge confirms presence of cross-reactivity and is consistent with a nonimmunologic type of reaction.
- A negative ASA challenge excludes cross-reactivity and is strongly supportive of an immunologic reaction to the single NSAID which caused the past adverse reaction.

In the case that ASA is the culprit drug, the patient can be challenged with an alternative strong COX-1 inhibitor (ie, ibuprofen) with similar conclusions based on a positive or negative challenge result.

## MANAGEMENT OF HYPERSENSITIVITY REACTIONS TO NONSTEROIDAL ANTIINFLAMMATORY DRUGS

Various options are available to successfully manage NSAID hypersensitivity. Nonetheless, all decisions depend on the correct identification of the type of reaction the patient experienced. If the reaction type is unclear, it is always best to have the patient strictly avoid all NSAIDs until additional evaluation can be performed by a drug allergy specialist.

Pharmacologic treatment options, listed by reaction subtype, are presented in this section. As a general rule, the best option for the affected patient is contingent upon their antiinflammatory and/or pain relief requirements.

**Table 3**
Oral ASA/NSAID challenge protocols based on suspected subtype of NSAID hypersensitivity reaction

| Suspected Subtype of NSAID Hypersensitivity Reactions | NSAID-Exacerbated Asthma and Rhinosinusitis (AERD)[a] | NECD/NIUA[b] | Mixed NSAID-Induced Reactions | Single NSAID-Induced Urticaria/Angioedema[c] | Single NSAID-Induced anaphylaxis[c] |
|---|---|---|---|---|---|
| Starting dose of ASA (mg) | 40.5 | 40.5 | 40.5 | 162 | 162 |
| Amount of ASA increased per step[d] | Double prior dose | Double prior dose | Double prior dose | Double prior dose | Double prior dose |
| Interval time between steps | 3 h | 90 min | 90 min | 3 h | 3 h |
| Common reaction doses (mg) | 60–100 | 162–650 | 60–100 | — | — |

*Abbreviations:* AERD, aspirin exacerbated-respiratory disease; ASA, aspirin; NECD, NSAID-exacerbated cutaneous disease; NIUA, NSAID-induced urticaria/angioedema; NSAID, nonsteroidal antiinflammatory drug.

[a] Patients should be pretreated with leukotriene modifying drug (ie, montelukast) and inhaled corticosteroid/long-acting beta-agonist combination (ICS/LABA) before challenge. ASA challenge is to determine whether patients are sensitive to ASA and might benefit from continuous daily ASA therapy. This is not a desensitization protocol.

[b] If ASA is required for cardiovascular protection, challenge can stop once patient reaches 81 mg without reaction. However, consider challenging to full 325 mg dose to confirm lack of persistent sensitivity to ASA because NSAID-exacerbated cutaneous disease (NECD) patients can often tolerate 81 mg but not full-strength ASA/NSAID.

[c] Culprit NSAID should be avoided. ASA or other NSAID (structurally unrelated to the culprit drug) should be used during the challenge. These patients are challenged to rule out presence of a nonimmunologic reaction; therefore, symptom onset is not expected.

[d] The challenge is stopped when the patient has a reaction or the desired therapeutic dose is reached.

### Nonimmunologic Hypersensitivity Reactions

#### Acetaminophen (paracetamol)
This is the simplest, and most likely cost-effective, option as long as the patient does not require an antiinflammatory pain reliever. Acetaminophen is generally well-tolerated at up to 650 mg per dose.[25] At higher doses (ie, 1000 mg), patients may experience untoward reactions owing to weak COX-1 inhibition that is induced at these doses.

#### Weak cyclooxygenase-1 inhibitors
This is a valuable choice for patients who desire antiinflammatory treatment, on the condition that they get adequate pain relief from these low potency NSAIDs. As with acetaminophen, these drugs may inhibit COX-1 at higher doses. If the patient's historical reaction to an NSAID was severe, some experts suggest administering the first dose (or the highest dose the patient is expected to tolerate) in a medically supervised setting.

#### Weak cyclooxygenase-2 inhibitors
There are few data on the use of these agents in patients with nonimmunologic NSAID hypersensitivity reactions. Therefore, they should be strictly avoided or given for the first time in a medically supervised setting.

#### Selective cyclooxygenase-2 inhibitors
With few exceptions, these are well-tolerated by patients and an excellent option for those who require strong antiinflammatory or pain reliever treatment. Additionally, this is a favorable option for patients who have experienced GI side effects from NSAID therapy. It is generally recommended that patients start at a low dose of the medication and gradually increase the dose as tolerated, particularly in those with AERD.

### Immunologic Hypersensitivity Reactions

Given the IgE-mediated nature of these reactions and subsequent risk for anaphylaxis, all patients with these types of reactions should strictly avoid the culprit NSAID. As mentioned, if there is any uncertainty regarding the type of reaction the patient experienced, a drug challenge with ASA (under the guidance of an allergy specialist) should be considered to definitely exclude a nonimmunologic reaction. Once the diagnosis is confirmed, patients may safely take NSAIDs that are chemically dissimilar to the drug that caused the initial reaction (see **Box 1**). Desensitization to the culprit NSAID is not recommended given the risk of the procedure and availability of other COX-1 inhibitors for any necessary antiinflammatory treatment.

### Desensitization

If the patient has undergone a positive oral challenge and requires chronic NSAID therapy, the clinician may elect to pursue NSAID desensitization to induce tolerance to the drug. The process of desensitization is essentially a continuation of the challenge protocol until the patient reaches the desired dose of the medication and has no further adverse reactions. Of the various nonimmunologic reaction subtypes, AERD responds most favorably to desensitization (see Waldram JD, Simon RA: Performing Aspirin Desensitization in Aspirin Exacerbated Respiratory Disease, in this issue). It has shown mixed results with the other forms of nonimmunologic reactions and is generally unsuccessful for patients with NECD. It is not recommended for affected patients with immunologic reactions owing to the potential risk of inducing anaphylaxis during the procedure.

## SUMMARY

NSAIDs are among the most common causes of ADRs worldwide. Symptoms of NSAID sensitivity range from predictable side effects to life-threatening anaphylaxis. The ability to appropriately diagnose and categorize these reactions is crucial. Our understanding of both the immunologic and nonimmunologic mechanisms of these reactions, along with the pharmaceutical development of selective COX-2 inhibitors, has greatly influenced our ability to successfully manage these patients.

## REFERENCES

1. Wilcox CM, Cryer B, Triadafilopoulos G. Patterns of use and public perception of over-the-counter pain relievers: focus on nonsteroidal antiinflammatory drugs. J Rheumatol 2005;32(11):2218–24.

2. Howard RL, Avery AJ, Slavenburg S, et al. Which drugs cause preventable admissions to hospital? A systematic review. Br J Clin Pharmacol 2007;63:136.

3. Vane JR. Inhibition of prostaglandin synthesis as a mechanism of action for aspirin-like drugs. Nat New Biol 1971;231:232.

4. Meade EA, Smith WL, DeWitt DL. Differential inhibition of prostaglandin endoperoxide synthase (cyclooxygenase) isozymes by aspirin and other non-steroidal anti-inflammatory drugs. J Biol Chem 1993;268:6610–4.

5. Dubois RN, Abramson SB, Crofford L, et al. Cyclooxygenase in biology and disease. FASEB J 1998;12:1063.

6. Trelle S, Reichenbach S, Wandel S, et al. Cardiovascular safety of non-steroidal anti-inflammatory drugs: network meta-analysis. BMJ 2011;342:c708.

7. Nissen SE. Cox-2 inhibitors and cardiovascular disease: considerable heat, but not much light. Eur Heart J 2012;33(21):2631–3.

8. Stevenson DD, Sanchez-Borges M, Szczeklik A. Classification of allergic and pseudoallergic reactions to drugs that inhibit cyclooxygenase enzymes. Ann Allergy Asthma Immunol 2001;87:177–80.

9. Kowalski ML, Makowska JS, Blanca M, et al. Hypersensitivity to nonsteroidal anti-inflammatory drugs (NSAIDs) – classification, diagnosis and management re: review of the EAACI/ENDA and GA2LEN/HANNA. Allergy 2011;66:818–29.

10. Kowalski ML, Asero R, Bavbek S, et al. Classification and practical approach to the diagnosis and management of hypersensitivity to nonsteroidal anti-inflammatory drugs. Allergy 2013;68:1219–32.

11. Morales DR, Guthrie B, Lipworth BJ, et al. NSAID-exacerbated respiratory disease: a meta-analysis evaluating prevalence, mean provocative dose of aspirin and increased asthma morbidity. Allergy 2015;70(7):828–35.

12. Woessner KM, Simon RA, Stevenson DD. The safety of celecoxib in patients with aspirin-sensitive asthma. Arthritis Rheum 2002;46:2201–6.

13. Sanchez-Borges M, Caballero-Fonseca F, Capriles-Hulett A, et al. Aspirin-exacerbated cutaneous disease (AECD) is a distinct subphenotype of chronic spontaneous urticaria. J Eur Acad Dermatol Venereol 2015;29(4):698–701.

14. Mathison DA, Lumry WR, Stevenson DD, et al. Aspirin in chronic urticaria and/or angioedema: studies of sensitivity and desensitization. J Allergy Clin Immunol 1982;69:135.

15. Doña I, Blanca-López N, Jagemann LR, et al. Response to a selective COX-2 inhibitor in patients with urticaria/angioedema induced by nonsteroidal anti-inflammatory drugs. Allergy 2011;66:1428–33.

16. Leeyaphan C, Kulthanan K, Jongjarearnprasert K, et al. Drug-induced angioedema without urticaria: prevalence and clinical features. J Eur Acad Dermatol Venereol 2010;24:685–91.

17. Sanchez-Borges M, Acevedo N, Caraballo L, et al. Increased total and mite specific immunoglobulin E in patients with aspirin-induced urticaria and angioedema. J Investig Allergol Clin Immunol 2010;20:139–45.

18. Doña I, Blanca-López N, Torres MJ, et al. NSAID-induced urticaria/angioedema does not evolve into chronic urticaria: a 12-year follow-up study. Allergy 2014; 69:438–44.

19. Doña I, Blanca-López N, Cornejo-Garcia JA, et al. Characteristics of subjects experiencing hypersensitivity to non-steroidal anti-inflammatory drugs: patterns of response. Clin Exp Allergy 2011;41:86–95.

20. Zembowicz A, Mastalerz L, Setkowicz M, et al. Histological spectrum of cutaneous reactions to aspirin in chronic idiopathic urticaria. J Cutan Pathol 2004; 31:323–9.

21. Woessner KM, Castells M. NSAID single-drug induced reactions. Immunol Allergy Clin N Am 2013;33(2):237–49.

22. Quiralte J, Blanco C, Castillo R, et al. Anaphylactoid reactions due to nonsteroidal antiinflammatory drugs: clinical and cross-reactivity studies. Ann Allergy Asthma Immunol 1997;78(3):293–6.

23. Picaud J, Beaudouin E, Renaudin JM, et al. Anaphylaxis to diclofenac: nine cases reported to the Allergy Vigilance Network in France. Allergy 2014;69(10):1420–3.

24. Kowalski ML, Bienkiewicz B, Woszczek G, et al. Diagnosis of pyrazolone drug sensitivity: clinical history versus skin testing and in vitro testing. Allergy Asthma Proc 1999;20:347–52.

25. Settipane RA, Schrank PJ, Simon RA, et al. Prevalence of cross-reactivity with acetaminophen in aspirin-sensitive asthmatic subjects. J Allergy Clin Immunol 1995;96:480.

26. Levy MB, Fink JN. Anaphylaxis to celecoxib. Ann Allergy Asthma Immunol 2001; 87:72.

27. Fontaine C, Bousquet PJ, Demoly P. Anaphylactic shock caused by a selective allergy to celecoxib, with no allergy to rofecoxib or sulfamethoxazole. J Allergy Clin Immunol 2005;115:633.

28. Gebhardt M, Wollina U. Cutaneous side-effects of nonsteroidal anti-inflammatory drugs (NSAID). Z Rheumatol 1995;54:405–12.

29. Patel RM, Marfatia YS. Clinical study of cutaneous drug eruptions in 200 patients. Indian J Dermatol Venereol Leprol 2008;74:430.

30. Ward KE, Archambault R, Mersfelder TL. Severe adverse skin reactions to nonsteroidal antiinflammatory drugs: a review of the literature. Am J Health Syst Pharm 2010;67:206–13.

31. Mockenhaupt M, Kelly JP, Kaufman D, et al, SCAR Study Group. The risk of Stevens-Johnson syndrome and toxic epidermal necrolysis associated with nonsteroidal antiinflammatory drugs: a multinational perspective. J Rheumatol 2003;30:2234–40.

32. Mihovilovic K, Ljubanovic D, Knotek M. Safe administration of celecoxib to a patient with repeated episodes of nephrotic syndrome induced by NSAIDs. Clin Drug Investig 2011;31:351–5.

33. Kowalski ML, Makowska JS. Seven steps to the diagnosis of NSAIDs hypersensitivity: how to apply a new classification in real practice? Allergy Asthma Immunol Res 2015;7(4):312–20.

34. Doña I, Blanca-López N, Torres MJ, et al. Drug hypersensitivity reactions: response patterns, drug involved, and temporal variations in a large series of patients. J Investig Allergol Clin Immunol 2012;22:363–71.
35. Stevens W, Buchheit K, Cahill KN. Aspirin-exacerbated diseases: advances in asthma with nasal polyposis, urticaria, angioedema, and anaphylaxis. Curr Allergy Asthma Rep 2015;15:69.
36. Palma-Carlos AG, Medina M, Palma-Carlos ML. Skin tests in NSAIDs hypersensitivity. Eur Ann Allergy Clin Immunol 2006;38(6):182–5.
37. Blanca-López N, Torres MJ, Doña I, et al. Value of the clinical history in the diagnosis of urticaria/angioedema induced by NSAIDs with cross-tolerance. Clin Exp Allergy 2013;43:85–91.
38. Viola M, Rumi G, Valluzzi RL, et al. Assessing potential determinants of positive provocation tests in subjects with NSAID hypersensitivity. Clin Exp Allergy 2011;41:96–103.
39. White AA, Stevenson DD, Woessner KM, et al. Approach to patients with aspirin hypersensitivity and acute cardiovascular emergencies. Allergy Asthma Proc 2013;34:138–42.

# Clinical Characteristics of Aspirin-Exacerbated Respiratory Disease

Donald D. Stevenson, MD, Andrew A. White, MD*

## KEYWORDS

- Aspirin • Nonsteroidal anti-inflammatory drugs • Nasal polyposis • Quality of life
- Asthma • Chronic rhinosinusitis • Cyclooxygenase 1

## KEY POINTS

- Aspirin-exacerbated respiratory disease presents with characteristic features of adult-onset nasal polyposis, asthma, and hypersensitivity reactions to aspirin or other nonsteroidal anti-inflammatory drugs.
- Aspirin-exacerbated respiratory disease is present in about 7% of all asthmatics and represents a phenotype of more severe sinus disease and asthma.
- Features that suggest a diagnosis of aspirin-exacerbated respiratory disease include severe sinus inflammation on imaging, significant polyp recurrence postoperatively, marked anosmia, and alcohol intolerance.
- There continue to be unmet needs in caring for patients with aspirin-exacerbated respiratory disease. Aspirin is an effective treatment for many, but further treatment options are sought by the patient community.

## INTRODUCTION, HISTORICAL NOTES, AND NOMENCLATURE

Aspirin-exacerbated respiratory disease (AERD) was first described in a 1922 French publication by Professors Widal, Abrami, and Lenmoyes.[1] Although only a single case report, their 37-year-old female patient was admitted to the hospital for extensive oral challenges over several weeks. Their description of the patient included all the clinical features of AERD. The patient acquired the disease in her 20s and was plagued by nasal polyposis and asthma, and during oral challenges with tiny quantities of aspirin and antipyrine (the first nonaspirin nonsteroidal anti-inflammatory drug), experienced severe asthma attacks, hives, and rhinorrhea. Oral challenges with non–cyclooxygenase 1 (COX-1)-inhibiting drugs, such as chlorohydrate, urotropine, quinine, and pyramidon,

Scripps Clinic, Division of Allergy, Asthma and Immunology, 3811 Valley Centre Drive S99, San Diego, CA 92130, USA
* Corresponding author. Division of Allergy, Asthma and Immunology, Scripps Clinic, 3811 Valley Centre Drive S99, San Diego, CA 92130.
E-mail address: white.andrew@scrippshealth.org

Immunol Allergy Clin N Am 36 (2016) 643–655
http://dx.doi.org/10.1016/j.iac.2016.06.002
0889-8561/16/$ – see front matter © 2016 Elsevier Inc. All rights reserved.
immunology.theclinics.com

did not induce respiratory or cutaneous reactions. Not knowing any better, the doctors incorrectly called this disease *idiosyncratic anaphylaxis*. Actually, this 37-year-old woman had the first reported case of AERD.

Meanwhile, in the mid-1960s, Professor Max Samter, at the University of Chicago, also identified and described the same disease and, along with Professor Beers, published the first English description of AERD, which he called *aspirin intolerance or triad disease*. This disease then became known as *Samter's syndrome*.[2] At about the same time (1967), a report describing the first positive oral challenges with aspirin, and, on a separate occasion, indomethacin, in a patient with AERD, was published by Vanselow and Smith.[3] It was not until 1993 when Doctor Amy Klion translated Professor Widal's original 1922 case report from French into English,[4] that several investigators realized that Samter's syndrome was actually first described and reported in the literature by Professor Widal. Professors Samter and Beers emphasized and expanded the concept of cross-reactions to nonsteroidal anti-inflammatory drugs (NSAIDs).[5] Over the years, the preferred descriptor for this disease has wandered through a confusing list, including, in addition to Professor Samter's descriptions (intolerance and triad), *aspirin idiosyncrasy*, *aspirin-sensitive rhinosinusitis/asthma*, *aspirin-induced asthma*, *NSAID-induced asthma*, and, finally the 2 currently accepted descriptions, *AERD* in the United States and *NSAID-induced respiratory disease* in Europe. All of these terms describe the disease and not the reactions, which are generally called *acute hypersensitivity reactions to aspirin* (or any NSAID involved in the respiratory reactions).[6]

## CLINICAL PRESENTATION

Somewhere around age 30, typical viral respiratory infections develop in otherwise healthy individuals or those with prior allergic rhinitis or asthma. However, unlike the usual clearing of an upper respiratory infection in 2 to 4 weeks, nasal congestion persists.[7,8] Early-onset AERD patients frequently describe their course as, "my cold never went away." A viral infection is one likely culprit in the initiation of AERD. It is possible that after a viral-induced immunologic insult, either anti-inflammatory pathways fail to resolve or epigenetic changes occur, which leads to ongoing irreversible inflammation. Perhaps the virus infection leads to other secondary events such as *Staphylococcus aureas* colonization or other perturbations in the microbiome that could enhance the inflammatory milieu. The true sequence of events in the first few days and weeks of AERD is unfortunately still speculative. It should be pointed out, however, that virus infections are found to enhance type 2 inflammations.[9,10] Alternatively, it is possible that when AERD develops in a healthy individual, the early symptoms are so similar to a viral upper respiratory tract infection that a virus falsely bears the blame. Up to 50% of subjects report a viral illness at the onset AERD.[8] How many viral infections go unreported is of course unknown. Environmental factors such as second-hand cigarette smoke exposure, especially in childhood, seem to increase the risk of AERD development.[11] After AERD is established and begins to evolve, patients subsequently have progressive nasal congestion, anosmia, and eventually pansinusitis with nasal polyposis. In most patients, asthma joins the upper airway disease as the next pathologic event. At this point, patients look like any other person with pansinusitis and asthma. The difference is that a diagnosis of AERD requires both the presence of nasal polyps, sinusitis (and sometimes asthma), plus a respiratory reaction after ingestion of aspirin or any of the NSAIDs that inhibit COX-1. Only then, and not before, is the diagnosis of AERD secure. This NSAID ingestion event can occur at any time in the evolution of the disease.

The original conundrum that perplexed all thoughtful investigators has been, if aspirin causes reactions in the respiratory tract, why do these patients continue to have respiratory inflammation in the absence of ingesting any further aspirin or other NSAIDs? The answer seems to be that AERD is an inflammatory disease, characterized by continuous immune dysregulation. Inflammation continues and builds on itself or is augmented by other comorbid diseases. Its perpetuation and severity has nothing to do with the occasional hypersensitivity reactions to ingestion or injection of NSAIDs but rather to the sum and substance of the underlying AERD inflammatory syndrome plus any superimposed comorbid conditions. AERD patients, while avoiding aspirin and other NSAIDs, experience all events characteristic of chronic asthma. Viral respiratory infections, irritant exposure, gastroesophageal reflux, exercise, and IgE-mediated reactions to pollens, pets, foods, and dust mites all contribute to the clinical courses of patients with AERD. Underlying AERD neither protects nor excludes the contribution of other provoking mechanisms. Although most studies show that most AERD patients meet the criteria for severe asthma,[12] a spectrum of severity exists, from mild intermittent asthma with occasional use of albuterol inhaler to the most severe, corticosteroid-dependent asthmatic patients that physicians can ever encounter. Yet, some AERD patients do not have asthma at all but develop upper airway disease with negative methacholine inhalation challenges and oral aspirin challenges, which only induce upper airway reactions.[13]

## PREVALENCE OF ASPIRIN-EXACERBATED RESPIRATORY DISEASE

The true prevalence of AERD is probably unobtainable. As stated earlier, AERD consists of an underlying profile, shared by other inflammatory conditions, consisting of polypoid inflammation of the upper airway with or without asthma plus the hallmark event of acute hypersensitivity reactions to a COX-1–inhibiting drug, usually aspirin itself. It is this hallmark event that can be elusive because the historical reaction may only occur in the upper airway, has an average onset of 50 to 90 minutes after ingesting the inciting NSAID, may be mild, and relies on patient memory. Some patients never put the 2 events together in the first place (aspirin ingestion and 90 minutes later some respiratory symptoms). Alternatively, some patients ingest an NSAID, experience nasal or asthmatic symptoms in the next hour, and erroneously blame it on the aspirin, when it was caused by irritant fumes or an allergen. Furthermore, some physicians who have completed the process of diagnosing pansinusitis, nasal polyps, or asthma then warn their patients to avoid NSAIDs, including aspirin, for the rest of their life. Joining this cadre of NSAID-nonexposed patients is a sizable portion of the population that does not need NSAIDs or is perfectly happy taking low doses of acetaminophen and never takes an effective NSAID that has the potential of completing the last leg of the diagnostic criteria for AERD. Therefore, standard questionnaires of patients, asking whether they have AERD, are always inaccurate in identifying patients with AERD within a population of asthmatics, otherwise normal individuals, or those with rhinitis or pansinusitis.

Underdiagnosis of AERD can occur when conducting oral aspirin challenges in patients suspected of having AERD. The first problem stems from the dynamic nature of this disease. AERD is not standing still while an aspirin challenge test is conducted at one point in time. In fact, it is known that early on in the course of eventually correctly diagnosed AERD patients, historical and laboratory challenges with aspirin can be negative and only months later become positive as the disease evolves.[14] Second, with the introduction of leukotriene-modifying drugs, oral challenges with aspirin are modified[15,16] sometimes to the extent that oral challenges to aspirin are negative in patients who subsequently have a positive oral aspirin challenge after the leukotriene-modifying drug has been removed.[17] Therefore, even with provocative challenges with aspirin, overdiagnosis and underdiagnosis have occurred and will continue to occur, making the true prevalence of AERD elusive. Finally, some populations (China) seem to have a low prevalence of eosinophilic rhinosinusitis and AERD.[18] Most of the data on population studies was reported in Europe and the United States. This led to a wide variation in prevalence estimates for AERD, all of which require assessment of the underlying pitfalls outlined above. In an attempt to correct for these variables, our recent meta-analysis stratified for these potential biases by looking at study types separately and in aggregate. This study reported that the prevalence of AERD in the asthmatic population was 7.4%.[19] If asthmatics also have aggressive nasal polyps or pan sinusitis, the prevalence increased significantly to 25%.[20]

## DEMOGRAPHIC FEATURES

Most studies identify AERD slightly more commonly in women: as high as 2.3:1 ratio in a European cohort of 500 patients with AERD.[8] A similar US study found 57% women in a group of 300 AERD patients.[7] In the large European natural history study, women seemed to also have more severe disease.[8] This finding would be in line with those of other studies looking at gender effects in sinus disease and AERD.[21,22] In a large retrospective analysis of a single geographic population, there seemed to be an increased risk for AERD (odds ratio, 2.94) in African Americans when compared with white and Latino patients.[23] Little is known about the true heritability of AERD. In the 2 large natural history studies with a combined total of 800 subjects, the presence of AERD reported in a family member was 1% and 6%.[7,8]

## CROSS-REACTIONS WITH CYCLOOXYGENASE 1–INHIBITING MEDICATIONS

In 1975, Professor Szczeklik and colleagues[24] published the results of their landmark study on the mechanism of cross-reactions within the class of COX-1–inhibiting drugs. Dr. Szczeklik showed that drugs that inhibited microsomal prostaglandin synthetase in vitro (aspirin, indomethacin, mefenamic acid, flufenamic acid, and phenylbutazone) also induced acute asthma exacerbations in 11 volunteer AERD patients. By contrast, therapeutic doses of salicylamide, paracetamol (acetaminophen), benzydamine, and chloroquine, which did not inhibit prostaglandins, did not induced asthmatic reactions in the same AERD volunteers. These early studies have been reproduced and expanded over the years. However, the principles of COX-1 (prostaglandin synthetase) inhibition initiating cross-reactivity have persisted to the present. Efficient inhibitors of COX-1 induce strong asthmatic reactions and weak inhibitors of COX-1–induced mild reactions. If the drug does not inhibit COX-1 at all, it cannot and does not cross-react with aspirin in patients with AERD.

### Effective Cyclooxygenase 1 Inhibitors

The most commonly implicated NSAIDs causing the historical respiratory reaction were aspirin (80%), ibuprofen (41%), naproxen (4%), and ketorolac (1%).[7,8] In some patients, more than one respiratory reaction occurred, sometimes to 2 different NSAIDs (**Table 1**).

### Weak Cyclooxygenase 1 Inhibitors

Acetaminophen (paracetamol in Europe), when given in lower doses <500 mg, generally does not induce respiratory reactions in AERD patients. However, in doses >1000 mg, and up to 1500 mg, about one-third of AERD patients had mild

| Table 1 Effective COX-1 inhibitors | |
|---|---|
| **Generic Names** | **Brand Names** |
| Acetylsalicylic acid | Aspirin |
| Benoxaprofen | Oraflex |
| Diclofenac | Voltaren |
| Diflunisal | Dolobid |
| Etodolac | Lodine |
| Fenoprofen | Nalfon |
| Flurbiprofen | Ansaid |
| Ibuprofen | Motrin, Advil, Rufen |
| Indomethacin | Indocin |
| Ketoprofen | Orudis, Oruvail |
| Ketorolac | Toradol |
| Meclofenamate | Meclomen |
| Metamizole | Pyralginum |
| Mefenamic acid | Ponstel |
| Nabumetone | Relafen |
| Naproxen | Naprosyn, Aleve, Anaprox |
| Oxaprozin | Daypro |
| Piroxicam | Feldene |
| Tolmetin | Tolectin |

asthmatic and nasal reactions.[25] Salsalate, a weak inhibitor of COX-1, required high doses to induce minimal respiratory reactions.[26] One of the peculiarities of AERD cross-reactors is that only acetyl-salicylate (aspirin) efficiently inhibits COX-1 enzymes. The other salicylates are either weak inhibitors or, as exemplified by sodium salicylate, do not inhibit COX-1 at all and, therefore, do not cross-react with aspirin and the efficient NSAIDs.

### Partially Selective Cyclooxygenase 2 Inhibitors

Meloxicam and nimesulide are preferential COX-2 inhibitors when ingested at lower doses. However, at higher therapeutic doses, 15 mg for meloxicam for example, mild respiratory reactions in AERD patients were observed in a minority of patients.[27]

### Selective Cyclooxygenase 2 Inhibitors

These drugs are too large to fit in the smaller COX-1 channel and, therefore, cannot competitively inhibit COX-1. With COX-1 enzymes still operative, prostaglandin E2 is not depleted, and the respiratory reactions cannot occur. Two manufacturing companies withdrew rofecoxib and valdecoxib from the market. In the United States, only celecoxib is available by prescription. In the rest of the world, etoricoxib, lumiracoxib, and parecoxib are available and are safely prescribed for patients with AERD.

### The Yellow Dye Story

Professor Samter believed that tartrazine, also known as *Yellow Dye #5*, cross-reacted with aspirin in AERD patients and provided a stimulus for ongoing asthma because of daily ingestion of yellow-colored medications.[5] His theory turned out to be incorrect when more rigorous oral challenges were conducted. Tartrazine challenges, conducted in hundreds of AERD patients, were completely negative.[28,29] Sulfites, monosodium glutamate, and other azo dyes were also implicated as cross-reactors in the older literature. None of these molecules meet the criteria of being COX-1 inhibitors and are found to not cross-react with aspirin in patients with AERD.[26,30]

## CLINICAL REACTIONS TO CYCLOOXYGENASE 1 INHIBITION

The hallmark of AERD is the hypersensitivity reaction to aspirin and NSAIDS. Patients report these reactions 50 to 90 minutes after ingestion of a COX-1 inhibitor. During oral aspirin challenges, with 60 mg of aspirin, as the average provoking dose, the mean elapsed time from aspirin ingestion to start of respiratory symptoms was 102 minutes.[31] The difference between observed latency in the clinic during oral challenges and patient reports might be recall bias or the difference in doses between the 2 experiences (full therapeutic doses of 650 mg vs threshold doses of 60 mg). Reactions nearly always include respiratory symptoms, although these might be secondary in severity to gastrointestinal or cutaneous symptoms. Most patients have upper airway reactions (nasal congestion, sneezing, and ocular tearing and itching) with some experiencing lower respiratory symptoms of wheeze, shortness of breath, and a drop in forced expiratory values in first second of expiration ($FEV_1$) values. Although much less common, a distinct phenotype of clinical reactions has been described with symptoms predominantly in the gastrointestinal tract (nausea, vomiting, abdominal pain) with urticaria and flushing.[32] These reactions, particularly severe bronchospasm, can produce significant morbidity and occasionally mortality. Only 30% of acute reactions are adequately controlled at home. Most reactions (70%) require acute medical care—69% treated and released from the emergency room and 31% transitioned to hospitalization.[33]

## SEVERITY OF THE UNDERLYING DISEASE

In medical studies on patients with AERD, the severity of the disease is frequently diluted to a single known metric, for example, frequency of nasal polyp surgery or quality measures of asthma control. Yet, the effects of AERD are not one dimensional. Many patients suffer from sinus disease, asthma, and deprivation of NSAID treatment in the face of diseases that require these drugs. As such, there are no validated tools to measure the many domains of morbidity associated with AERD. Yet, when looking at the individual components of morbidity in AERD, several themes emerge.

### Aspirin-Exacerbated Respiratory Disease Patients Suffer from Accelerated Sinus Inflammation

Unusually severe polypoid disease invading the brain or perforating the tympanic membrane and erupting into the external auditory canal have been described in AERD patients.[34,35] The mechanisms of differences between AERD and non-AERD sinus inflammation are discussed in other articles in this issue, but, in general, the parameters of eosinophilic inflammation and mast cell activity are greater in AERD than in other forms of sinus disease. Therefore, in AERD, this condition leads to increased use of medications with higher use of systemic corticosteroids and markedly increased need for sinus revision surgery. The degree of inflammation on computed tomography sinus imaging correlates significantly with the likelihood of having AERD.[36] Patients with AERD are likely to have up to 10-fold the number of sinus surgeries as aspirin-tolerant patients and more likely to have recurrence by 6 months.[20]

When looking at the 22-item Sinonasal Outcome Test (SNOT-22), a validated assessment of chronic rhinosinusitis, AERD was only clustered in the severe and moderate sinonasal scores, with no AERD patients in the mild (SNOT-22 score, 16) group.[37] In this study, the severe group (SNOT-22 score, 90.8), enriched for AERD, was more likely to have rapid relapses postoperatively. In that the epicenter of the disease in AERD is the sinus mucosa, sinus disease is expected to cause much of the morbidity in AERD. The repeated sinus surgeries have their own morbidity, with associated high economic costs. The disease lends itself to patient misery with loss of sense of smell and frequent sinus infections. AERD patients average 5.5 superimposed viral/bacterial sinus infections per year.[7] In a recent survey of AERD patients, which ranked how severe AERD affected quality of life, the average score was 6 (1, mild; 9, severe).[38] The 2 most common domains affecting their quality of life were chronic nasal symptoms (87%) and decreased sense of smell (89%). The effect of these symptoms on overall quality of life is likely eclipsed in medical studies by the easier-to-study endpoints of asthma exacerbation, corticosteroid bursts, emergency room visits, and need for revision sinus surgery.

### Asthma Morbidity and Mortality Are Frequently a Part of Aspirin-Exacerbated Respiratory Disease

Although asthma is not an essential component of the disease, when present, it is often more severe than asthma found in aspirin-tolerant asthmatics. The best evidence for this finding comes from the Tenor study but can also be seen in other severe asthma cohorts, which are frequently enriched for AERD.[12,39,40] Death from status asthmaticus can occur during an NSAID-induced asthma exacerbation or during a viral infection, when no NSAIDs are ingested.[41] In a European study, only 20.4% of AERD patients had controlled asthma, and 45.3% of asthmatics were rated as uncontrolled. Higher baseline $FEV_1$ values, lack of airway reversibility, and referral to a specialty center were factors associated with better asthma control.[42] A recent meta-analysis evaluated asthma morbidity in 7 studies. This analysis found that in AERD, asthma was uncontrolled in 18.9% compared with 10.4% of aspirin-tolerant asthmatics. In AERD, 59.4% had asthma categorized as severe when compared with 38.7% of control asthmatics. This study determined that the risk of emergency care for asthma was increased by 80% in AERD, the risk of asthma hospitalization increased by 40%, and the rate of outpatient asthma exacerbations was increased by 60% when compared with aspirin-tolerant asthmatics.[39] These data underscore that when asthma is present in AERD, it is frequently labile and severe.

### Perceived Effectiveness of Medical Treatment in AERD

Among a large group of AERD patients, daily aspirin therapy, after desensitization, was felt to be the most effective treatment in those that received this intervention.[38] Of the general population of AERD patients, 35% did not feel that any medication was effective. Yet, of this group, 81% had never been desensitized to aspirin and then treated with daily aspirin therapy. This finding argues that aspirin therapy is not offered by physicians or, if offered, is not desired by a significant percent of AERD patients. These findings present an opportunity for improvement in the future. Aspirin therapy is found to be beneficial for most patients with AERD, but approximately 15% discontinue therapy because of side effects, and another 15% obtain no benefit.[43] Although several potentially beneficial monoclonal antibodies are in phase 2 to 3 studies for asthma and sinus disease, none are specifically undergoing studies in patients with AERD.

## ALCOHOL REACTIVITY IN ASPIRIN-EXACERBATED RESPIRATORY DISEASE PATIENTS

Respiratory reactions to alcohol have been reported in the literature for nearly 15 years, yet it is few aspirin-tolerant asthmatic subjects who report respiratory reactions to alcohol.[44,45] These reactions are characterized by typical asthmatic symptoms of cough, wheeze, and chest tightness, not the flushing seen in some Asian individuals who lack the acetaldehyde dehydrogenase enzyme. A recent survey identified specific respiratory reactions in most AERD patients.[46] This not only included chest symptoms of cough and wheeze but also rhinitis symptoms of congestion and rhinorrhea. These reactions can be immediate and uncomfortable enough that many AERD patients stop drinking alcohol entirely. The mechanics of this reactivity are unclear, but a COX-1 inhibition mechanism is not plausible for several reasons. The most conclusive evidence for a non–COX-1 mechanism is the persistence of alcohol reactivity even after aspirin desensitization. Reactions to alcohol can occur with any type of alcohol, arguing against a specific component of alcohol such as sulfites, tannins, and hops. Some evidence suggests that the target organ (upper airway vs lower airway) during aspirin reactions is similar to the target of alcohol reactions.[46] Yet, although much more common in AERD, the reactivity to alcohol is not specific for AERD. Upper airway reactions occur in aspirin-tolerant sinus disease and asthma, albeit at lower frequency than seen in AERD. In a mouse model of allergic inflammation, ethanol gavage was able to immediately trigger airway mucin production and airway obstruction but only in sensitized mice, not in unsensitized mice.[47] Together these data suggest that alcohol augments or amplifies existent inflammation through a non–COX-1–mediated mechanism. The degree of underlying inflammation might need to be greater than a specific threshold for alcohol to trigger respiratory reactions. The finding that in certain individuals tolerance of alcohol occurs after aspirin desensitization could be explained in the context of an overall anti-inflammatory effect.[48]

## CONCOMITANT ATOPIC DISEASE

It is clear that the rate of atopic disease in AERD patients is higher than that in the general population.[7,8] However, at least one-third of known AERD patients have negative histories and negative skin test results to common aeroallergens, showing that AERD can evolve in the absence of IgE-mediated mucosal inflammation.[7] The presence of elevated serum IgE levels in skin test–negative individuals has been described in AERD. These subjects had no other defining characteristics, and the IgE level did not correlate with eosinophilia.[49] Interestingly, in a study of asthma severity in AERD, serum IgE levels were correlated with asthma severity but not with positive skin testing.[42] It should be noted that high levels of IgE to Staphylococcal super antigens in AERD patients, a potential cause of ongoing mucosal inflammation, have been associated with higher total IgE, airway hyper-responsiveness, eosinophil activation, and more severe clinical symptoms.[50] In a large group of AERD patients, after treatment with aspirin desensitization, a subgroup of 16 aspirin nonresponders was identified. In this group, clinically relevant atopic disease was identified. The authors argued that allergic disease can be a comorbid provocateur in AERD and should be treated as such.[43] To date, there is no evidence that atopy influences the risk of AERD development. However, the presence of atopy can augment the level of inflammation as a comorbid condition.

## HETEROGENEITY WITHIN THE DISEASE OF ASPIRIN-EXACERBATED RESPIRATORY DISEASE

Although AERD has several typical features, heterogeneity within AERD does exist. Bochenek and colleagues[21] used a latent class analysis method to segregate certain features of AERD. Their results identified 4 subtypes of AERD:

- Class 1 contained moderate asthmatics, severe sinus disease, and blood eosinophilia.
- Class 2 exhibited mild rhinosinusitis, mild asthma, and low health care utilization.
- Class 3 featured severe asthmatics, prone to severe exacerbations and significant airway obstruction.
- Class 4 also comprised poorly controlled asthmatics but in contrast to Class 3, were exclusively female, had relatively normal lung function, and were much more likely to be obese.

Interestingly, atopy did not segregate into any of the 4 classes. Both class 3 and 4 were associated with high health care utilization, primarily related to uncontrolled asthma. These findings show that within AERD, there are differences in target organ involvement and in degree and persistence of the inflammation and thus disease severity.[21]

## PITFALLS AND DIAGNOSTIC DILEMMAS

According to the Centers for Disease Control, 1 in 12 Americans have asthma. If 7% of the 18.7 million adult asthmatics in the country have AERD, then 1.3 million AERD patients exist in the United States. Yet this disease continues to be overlooked by primary care internists and family practice physicians, chest physicians, head and neck surgeons, and allergists. **Box 1** shows several of the factors complicating the identification and proper disposition of these patients.

---

**Box 1**
**Diagnostic considerations in AERD**

*In favor of AERD*

Aggressive polyp formation

Complete anosmia

Alcohol intolerance (respiratory)

Severe inflammation seen on computed tomography scan of sinuses

History of respiratory symptoms with COX-1 inhibitor

*Against AERD*

Mild sinus disease

No early polyp recurrence after surgery

Tolerance of alcohol

Recent tolerance of a COX-1 inhibitor

*Confounding Factors*

Chronic low-dose aspirin does not rule out AERD

Severe gastrointestinal reactions are likely to be AERD

Controlled aspirin challenges can be false-negative

First, it is clear that some patients may be taking daily low-dose NSAIDS and still have AERD.[51] If the clinical history suggests AERD, one should not be dissuaded by a history of daily NSAID use. This history almost always involves daily ingestion of aspirin, 81 mg, for prevention of vascular thrombosis. Many of these patients had such a minor respiratory reaction on the first day they took 81 mg of aspirin that they never noted or reported this as an unusual event. Physicians may not have asked critical questions about the first day of ingesting 81 mg of aspirin. Once they were taking aspirin daily, patients effectively desensitized themselves to aspirin and no longer experienced reactions each morning when they took their daily 81 mg of aspirin. Consideration should be made to withdraw aspirin and perform an oral aspirin challenge. Although 81 mg of aspirin each day can maintain a desensitized state, such a low dose rarely interrupts sinonasal inflammation.

Second, during oral aspirin challenges in de novo AERD patients, silent desensitization can occur.[17] In this situation, pretreatment with a leukotriene modifier, to protect the patient from a severe exacerbation of asthma, in combination with an escalating graded challenge, culminates in an oral aspirin challenge with no symptoms. Withdrawal of the protective leukotriene blocker and repeated challenges are diagnostic in patients with true AERD.

Third, patient histories of NSAID tolerance or reactivity are not specific or sensitive enough to exclude AERD. Between 10% and 15% of patients, ultimately proven to have AERD after a diagnostic aspirin challenge, had no known history of reactivity to aspirin or an NSAID.[8] Conversely, some individuals (10%–15%) with sinus disease and asthma, who reported an association between ingestion of aspirin or other NSAIDs and an asthma attack, proceeded to negative aspirin challenges.[16]

Fourth, apathy on the part of an investigating physician can hinder any further diagnostic considerations. An aspirin challenge might be considered too complicated and referral to a specialist who can perform aspirin challenges, too much trouble. Daily treatment with aspirin, in the face of limited knowledge, might be viewed with skepticism followed by a "why does it matter" attitude on the part of some physicians. Thus, the opportunity to improve the lives of 1.3 million Americans who are afflicted with AERD is denied through misunderstanding and inattention.

## SUMMARY

AERD is a perplexing inflammatory airway disease. But it is only perplexing insofar as the initial inflammatory trigger is obscure, and the susceptibility to COX-1 inhibition still remains somewhat difficult to reconcile with our understanding of normal protective functions of prostaglandin E2. What is not difficult to identify is the clinical progression of AERD, of which, the characteristics in aggregate are typical and frequently easy to segregate diagnostically. The development of adult-onset nasal polyposis, which is recalcitrant to medical therapy and requires frequent surgical debulking in an individual who is either avoiding NSAIDS or has a history of NSAID-induced reactions, should immediately trigger a diagnosis of AERD unless properly excluded by a controlled negative NSAID challenge. It is clear that the diagnosis of AERD should not be exclusively dependent on a history of an NSAID-associated respiratory event, as these are not identified during oral aspirin challenges in up to 15% of AERD subjects.[8]

AERD remains a distinct endotype of both asthma and chronic sinusitis, important because of significant morbidity when compared with aspirin-tolerant forms of similar underlying diseases. The lack of a specific mechanism to explain the onset and perpetuation of AERD requires intensive research to design and test targeted therapies. In the meantime, the study of potential therapeutics in a disease for which additional therapeutic modalities are highly anticipated by the patient community requires ongoing support by the clinical and research communities. Aspirin desensitization and daily aspirin treatment are available now but are significantly underutilized.

## REFERENCES

1. Widal F, Abrami P, Lermoyez J. Anaphylaxie et idiosyncrasie. Presse Med 1922; 30:189–93.
2. Samter M, Beers RF Jr. Concerning the nature of intolerance to aspirin. J Allergy 1967;40(5):281–93.
3. Vanselow NA, Smith JR. Bronchial asthma induced by indomethacin. Ann Intern Med 1967;66(3):568–72.
4. Klion A. Widal on the aspirin triad and induction of tolerance. Allergy Asthma Proc 1993;14:371–2.
5. Samter M, Beers RF. Intolerance to aspirin. Clinical studies and consideration of its pathogenesis. Ann Intern Med 1968;68(5):975–83.
6. Kowalski ML, Makowska JS, Blanca M, et al. Hypersensitivity to nonsteroidal anti-inflammatory drugs (NSAIDs) - classification, diagnosis and management: review of the EAACI/ENDA and GA2LEN/HANNA. Allergy 2011;66(7):818–29.
7. Berges-Gimeno MP, Simon RA, Stevenson DD. The natural history and clinical characteristics of aspirin-exacerbated respiratory disease. Ann Allergy Asthma Immunol 2002;89(5):474–8.
8. Szczeklik A, Nizankowska E, Duplaga M. Natural history of aspirin-induced asthma. AIANE Investigators. European Network on Aspirin-Induced Asthma. Eur Respir J 2000;16(3):432–6.
9. Liu J, Wu J, Qi F, et al. Natural helper cells contribute to pulmonary eosinophilia by producing IL-13 via IL-33/ST2 pathway in a murine model of respiratory syncytial virus infection. Int Immunopharmacol 2015;28(1):337–43.
10. Chung Y, Hong JY, Lei J, et al. Rhinovirus infection induces interleukin-13 production from CD11b-positive, M2-polarized exudative macrophages. Am J Respir Cell Mol Biol 2015;52(2):205–16.
11. Chang JE, Ding D, Martin-Lazaro J, et al. Smoking, environmental tobacco smoke, and aspirin-exacerbated respiratory disease. Ann Allergy Asthma Immunol 2012;108(1):14–9.
12. Mascia K, Haselkorn T, Deniz YM, et al. Aspirin sensitivity and severity of asthma: evidence for irreversible airway obstruction in patients with severe or difficult-to-treat asthma. J Allergy Clin Immunol 2005;116(5):970–5.
13. Lumry WR, Curd JG, Zeiger RS, et al. Aspirin-sensitive rhinosinusitis: the clinical syndrome and effects of aspirin administration. J Allergy Clin Immunol 1983; 71(6):580–7.
14. Pleskow WW, Stevenson DD, Mathison DA, et al. Aspirin-sensitive rhinosinusitis/ asthma: spectrum of adverse reactions to aspirin. J Allergy Clin Immunol 1983; 71(6):574–9.
15. White AA, Stevenson DD, Simon RA. The blocking effect of essential controller medications during aspirin challenges in patients with aspirin-exacerbated respiratory disease. Ann Allergy Asthma Immunol 2005;95(4):330–5.
16. White A, Ludington E, Mehra P, et al. Effect of leukotriene modifier drugs on the safety of oral aspirin challenges. Ann Allergy Asthma Immunol 2006;97(5):688–93.
17. White AA, Bosso JV, Stevenson DD. The clinical dilemma of "silent desensitization" in aspirin-exacerbated respiratory disease. Allergy Asthma Proc 2013; 34(4):378–82.

18. Fan YP, Feng SY, Xia WT, et al. Aspirin-exacerbated respiratory disease in China: a cohort investigation and literature review. Am J Rhinol Allergy 2012;26(1): E20–2.
19. Rajan JP, Wineinger NE, Stevenson DD, et al. Prevalence of aspirin-exacerbated respiratory disease among asthmatic patients: a meta-analysis of the literature. J Allergy Clin Immunol 2015;135(3):676–81.e1.
20. Kim JE, Kountakis SE. The prevalence of Samter's triad in patients undergoing functional endoscopic sinus surgery. Ear Nose Throat J 2007;86(7):396–9.
21. Bochenek G, Kuschill-Dziurda J, Szafraniec K, et al. Certain subphenotypes of aspirin-exacerbated respiratory disease distinguished by latent class analysis. J Allergy Clin Immunol 2014;133(1):98–103.e1-6.
22. Stevens WW, Peters AT, Suh L, et al. A retrospective, cross-sectional study reveals that women with CRSwNP have more severe disease than men. Immun Inflamm Dis 2015;3(1):14–22.
23. Mahdavinia M, Benhammuda M, Codispoti CD, et al. African American Patients With Chronic Rhinosinusitis Have a Distinct Phenotype of Polyposis Associated With Increased Asthma Hospitalization. J Allergy Clin Immunol Pract 2016. [Epub ahead of print].
24. Szczeklik A, Gryglewski RJ, Czerniawska-Mysik G. Relationship of inhibition of prostaglandin biosynthesis by analgesics to asthma attacks in aspirin-sensitive patients. Br Med J 1975;1(5949):67–9.
25. Settipane RA, Stevenson DD. Cross sensitivity with acetaminophen in aspirin-sensitive subjects with asthma. J Allergy Clin Immunol 1989;84(1):26–33.
26. Stevenson DD, Hougham AJ, Schrank PJ, et al. Salsalate cross-sensitivity in aspirin-sensitive patients with asthma. J Allergy Clin Immunol 1990;86(5):749–58.
27. Senna GE, Passalacqua G, Dama A, et al. Nimesulide and meloxicam are a safe alternative drugs for patients intolerant to nonsteroidal anti-inflammatory drugs. Eur Ann Allergy Clin Immunol 2003;35(10):393–6.
28. Stevenson DD, Simon RA, Lumry WR, et al. Adverse reactions to tartrazine. J Allergy Clin Immunol 1986;78(1 Pt 2):182–91.
29. Stevenson D. Tartrazine, Azo and Non-Azo Dyes. In: Metcalf D, Sampson H, Simon R, editors. Food allergy: adverse reactions to foods and food additives. 4th edition. Malden (MA): Blackwell Publishing Company; 2008. p. 377–85.
30. Woessner KM, Simon RA, Stevenson DD. Monosodium glutamate sensitivity in asthma. J Allergy Clin Immunol 1999;104(2 Pt 1):305–10.
31. Hope AP, Woessner KA, Simon RA, et al. Rational approach to aspirin dosing during oral challenges and desensitization of patients with aspirin-exacerbated respiratory disease. J Allergy Clin Immunol 2009;123(2):406–10.
32. Cahill KN, Bensko JC, Boyce JA, et al. Prostaglandin D(2): a dominant mediator of aspirin-exacerbated respiratory disease. J Allergy Clin Immunol 2015;135(1): 245–52.
33. Williams AN, Simon RA, Woessner KM, et al. The relationship between historical aspirin-induced asthma and severity of asthma induced during oral aspirin challenges. J Allergy Clin Immunol 2007;120(2):273–7.
34. Majithia A, Tatla T, Sandhu G, et al. Intracranial polyps in patients with Samter's triad. Am J Rhinol 2007;21(1):59–63.
35. Shen J, Peterson M, Mafee M, et al. Aural polyps in Samter's triad: case report and literature review. Otol Neurotol 2012;33(5):774–8.
36. Mascia K, Borish L, Patrie J, et al. Chronic hyperplastic eosinophilic sinusitis as a predictor of aspirin-exacerbated respiratory disease. Ann Allergy Asthma Immunol 2005;94(6):652–7.

37. Divekar R, Patel N, Jin J, et al. Symptom-based clustering in chronic rhinosinusitis relates to history of aspirin sensitivity and postsurgical outcomes. J Allergy Clin Immunol Pract 2015;3(6):934–40.e3.
38. Ta V, White AA. Survey-defined patient experiences with aspirin-exacerbated respiratory disease. J Allergy Clin Immunol Pract 2015;3(5):711–8.
39. Morales DR, Guthrie B, Lipworth BJ, et al. NSAID-exacerbated respiratory disease: a meta-analysis evaluating prevalence, mean provocative dose of aspirin and increased asthma morbidity. Allergy 2015;70(7):828–35.
40. Lee JH, Haselkorn T, Borish L, et al. Risk factors associated with persistent airflow limitation in severe or difficult-to-treat asthma: insights from the TENOR study. Chest 2007;132(6):1882–9.
41. Picado C, Castillo JA, Montserrat JM, et al. Aspirin-intolerance as a precipitating factor of life-threatening attacks of asthma requiring mechanical ventilation. Eur Respir J 1989;2(2):127–9.
42. Bochenek G, Szafraniec K, Kuschill-Dziurda J, et al. Factors associated with asthma control in patients with aspirin-exacerbated respiratory disease. Respir Med 2015;109(5):588–95.
43. Berges-Gimeno MP, Simon RA, Stevenson DD. Long-term treatment with aspirin desensitization in asthmatic patients with aspirin-exacerbated respiratory disease. J Allergy Clin Immunol 2003;111(1):180–6.
44. Vally H, Taylor ML, Thompson PJ. The prevalence of aspirin intolerant asthma (AIA) in Australian asthmatic patients. Thorax 2002;57(7):569–74.
45. Misso NL, Aggarwal S, Thompson PJ, et al. Increases in urinary 9alpha,11beta-prostaglandin f2 indicate mast cell activation in wine-induced asthma. Int Arch Allergy Immunol 2009;149(2):127–32.
46. Cardet JC, White AA, Barrett NA, et al. Alcohol-induced respiratory symptoms are common in patients with aspirin exacerbated respiratory disease. J Allergy Clin Immunol Pract 2014;2(2):208–13.
47. Bouchard JC, Kim J, Beal DR, et al. Acute oral ethanol exposure triggers asthma in cockroach allergen-sensitized mice. Am J Pathol 2012;181(3):845–57.
48. Calais CJ, Banks TA. Resolution of alcohol-induced respiratory symptoms following aspirin desensitization in aspirin-exacerbated respiratory disease. Ann Allergy Asthma Immunol 2015;114(5):429–30.
49. Johns CB, Laidlaw TM. Elevated total serum IgE in nonatopic patients with aspirin-exacerbated respiratory disease. Am J Rhinol Allergy 2014;28(4):287–9.
50. Yoo HS, Shin YS, Liu JN, et al. Clinical significance of immunoglobulin E responses to staphylococcal superantigens in patients with aspirin-exacerbated respiratory disease. Int Arch Allergy Immunol 2013;162(4):340–5.
51. Lee-Sarwar K, Johns C, Laidlaw TM, et al. Tolerance of daily low-dose aspirin does not preclude aspirin-exacerbated respiratory disease. J Allergy Clin Immunol Pract 2015;3(3):449–51.

# Diagnostic Evaluation in Aspirin-Exacerbated Respiratory Disease

Adam N. Williams, MD[a,b,*]

## KEYWORDS

- Aspirin-exacerbated respiratory disease • Diagnosis • NSAID hypersensitivity
- Chronic rhinosinusitis with nasal polyps • Asthma • Intranasal ketorolac
- Oral aspirin challenge • Lysine-aspirin

## KEY POINTS

- The diagnosis of aspirin-exacerbated respiratory disease (AERD) is based on the history and confirmed by nonsteroidal anti-inflammatory drug (NSAID) provocation challenge.
- Options for diagnostic challenge include lysine-aspirin challenge by intranasal or inhalation (not available in the United States), oral aspirin challenge, and intranasal ketorolac and modified oral aspirin challenge.
- Oral aspirin challenge is considered the gold standard for diagnosis of AERD.
- Positive provocation challenges result in respiratory and systemic reactions of varying degrees of severity requiring close monitoring and treatment.
- Positive provocation challenges are usually performed as the initial step to NSAID desensitization.

## INTRODUCTION

Aspirin-exacerbated respiratory disease (AERD) is widely accepted as a distinct clinical disease, characterized classically by the triad of chronic hyperplastic, eosinophil-rich rhinosinusitis with nasal polyps; asthma; and hypersensitivity reactions to inhibitors of cyclo-oxygenase 1 enzyme (COX-1), such as nonsteroidal anti-inflammatory drugs (NSAIDs). Distinguishing the clinical triad of AERD from other phenotypes of chronic rhinosinusitis with nasal polyps (CRSNP), asthma, and NSAID reactivity is very important for 2 main reasons.

First, patients with AERD are at risk of experiencing very distressing and even life-threatening reactions following ingestion of NSAIDs. In cases of uncertainty regarding

Disclosure Statement: Nothing to disclose.
[a] Department of Allergy, Asthma, and Immunology, Bend Memorial Clinic, 815 Southwest Bond Street, Bend, OR 97702, USA; [b] School of Medicine, Oregon Health and Sciences University, 3181 SW Sam Jackson Park Road, Portland, OR 97239, USA
* Bend Memorial Clinic, 815 Southwest Bond Street, Bend, OR 97702.
E-mail address: awilliams@bmctotalcare.com

Immunol Allergy Clin N Am 36 (2016) 657–668
http://dx.doi.org/10.1016/j.iac.2016.06.003          immunology.theclinics.com
0889-8561/16/$ – see front matter © 2016 Elsevier Inc. All rights reserved.

tolerance of NSAIDs, patients with AERD would need to be counseled that future ingestion of NSAIDs could result in serious reactions, whereas individuals with CRSNP and/or asthma who do not have AERD should not be unduly restricted from taking these NSAIDs when clinically indicated for anti-inflammatory, analgesic, or cardiovascular benefit.

Second, there are treatment modalities uniquely beneficial in patients with AERD as compared with other phenotypes of CRSNP and asthma. As noted elsewhere in this journal, treatment with antileukotriene therapy and long-term treatment with aspirin following aspirin desensitization can have significant therapeutic benefit in AERD.

Although establishing the diagnosis of AERD is important for a number of reasons, making an accurate diagnosis can be challenging. This article is intended to assist the clinician in using the medical history and clinically available diagnostic modalities to accurately identify those patients with AERD, so that they may benefit from the therapies useful in this condition.

## DIAGNOSTIC UTILITY OF THE CLINICAL PRESENTATION

The diagnosis of AERD is suggested based on the clinical presentation and confirmed when an individual with a history suggestive of AERD has a clinically observed reaction to aspirin or another NSAID administered by 1 of 3 routes: intranasal, inhalation, or oral ingestion (oral aspirin challenge [OAC]).

Awareness of the prevalence of AERD in patients with CRSNP and asthma can be helpful in the approach to diagnosing AERD. Estimates of the prevalence of AERD in individuals with asthma, CRSNP, or both vary widely depending on the disease severity and means of diagnosis. A recent meta-analysis of several epidemiologic studies found the prevalence of AERD in certain populations to be

- 7% asthma
- 15% severe asthma
- 10% nasal polyps
- 9% unspecified chronic rhinosinusitis[1]

Although the history is helpful in making the diagnosis of AERD, it should not be relied on exclusively. Many patients with AERD may not be aware of their NSAID hypersensitivity. The onset of the reaction can be delayed by 2 to 3 hours after NSAID ingestion, making it difficult for the patient to make the connection between NSAID ingestion and any sudden increase in respiratory symptoms. Some patients with CRSNP and asthma may not have an occasion to take NSAIDs after the onset of disease, whereas others may have been advised to avoid NSAIDs before NSAID intolerance is suggested or confirmed. A European study reported that 15% of patients confirmed to have AERD after a positive challenge were not aware of their NSAID hypersensitivity before challenge.[2]

Dursun and colleagues[3] examined the value of the history provided by the patient in the diagnosis of AERD. In this study involving 243 patients with asthma and CRSNP referred for OAC, prechallenge data were collected from patient recall and available medical records regarding the details of the clinical history, including number and severity of NSAID-induced reactions before presentation. Of the 12 patients who had always avoided NSAIDs, and therefore did not know if they could tolerate taking NSAIDs, 5 (42%) had a positive challenge. The chance of a positive OAC if the patient had at least 1 suspected NSAID reaction was 86%. Patients with 2 or more prior NSAID-induced reactions had an 89% chance of having a positive OAC. In patients with at least 1 severe reaction (defined as a poor response to albuterol and requiring medical intervention), 100% had a positive OAC result. In a multivariate analysis of several characteristics, the following were associated with a statistically significant higher likelihood of having a positive OAC:

- Multiple NSAID-induced reactions
- Age ≤40 years
- Poorer sense of smell[3]

## DIAGNOSTIC NONSTEROIDAL ANTI-INFLAMMATORY DRUG CHALLENGE

The diagnosis of AERD is confirmed with objectively observed signs of a hypersensitivity reaction provoked by graded inhalation, intranasal, or oral administration of NSAIDs. In Europe and other parts of the world, inhalation and intranasal provocation challenge testing has been widely available because of the availability of lysine-aspirin, a form of aspirin that is soluble and can therefore be administered in respirable droplets. In the United States, lysine-aspirin is not approved for use in humans by the US Food and Drug Administration. As a result, the only means of diagnostic provocation that had been available in the United States was provocation by oral challenge. In recent years, however, ketorolac tromethamine, an NSAID available in aqueous solution, has been used in intranasal challenge and is gaining wider acceptance and increasingly used in the diagnosis of AERD.[4,5]

OAC is considered the gold standard for confirming the diagnosis of AERD, with the greatest sensitivity.[6] **Table 1** lists the sensitivity and specificities of currently available provocation modalities. There are a number of variations of protocols for each type of diagnostic challenge technique that have been published and/or are in clinical use, limiting reliable comparisons in test performance.

### Indications and Contraindications for Diagnostic Challenge

The importance of diagnosing, or ruling out, AERD in patients with CRSNP and asthma cannot be overemphasized, as the implications for management are significant. Diagnostic NSAID challenge in patients with CRSNP and/or asthma is indicated in 2 main situations. First, it is used to determine NSAID tolerance status when it is not known. Many patients with CRSNP and/or asthma do not know whether they are able to tolerate NSAIDs, either because they are intentionally avoiding NSAIDs out of caution, have not had occasion to take NSAIDs, or have never temporally associated triggering of respiratory symptoms with taking NSAIDs.

Second, NSAID challenge is indicated to confirm the diagnosis of AERD in patients with CRSNP, asthma, and strongly suspected NSAID intolerance who have an indication for therapeutic use of NSAIDs, such as in the management of AERD, for cardiovascular benefit, or for anti-inflammatory or analgesic effects.

| Table 1 | | |
|---|---|---|
| Sensitivity and specificity of diagnostic challenges for aspirin-exacerbated respiratory disease | | |
| **Route of Challenge** | **Sensitivity, %** | **Specificity, %** |
| Oral | 89–90 | 93 |
| Bronchial | 77–90 | 93 |
| Intranasal | | |
|   Lysine-aspirin | 80–87 | 93–100 |
|   Ketorolac | 56–90 | 64–94 |

*Data from* Refs.[4,5,7–12]

## Contraindications for Diagnostic Challenge

NSAID challenges are considered contraindicated in patients with any of the following:

- History of severe anaphylactic reactions precipitated by aspirin or NSAIDs
- Unstable asthma
- Recent respiratory tract infection (within 4 weeks)
- Current pregnancy
- Severe underlying cardiovascular, renal, or liver disease[13]

Patients receiving therapy with beta-blockers may be at increased risk of more severe and difficult-to-treat reactions. Some guidelines consider beta-blockers to be a contraindication, whereas others recommend taking additional precautions in patients who are unable to stop taking them.[13,14]

## Preparation for Diagnostic Challenge

NSAID challenges should be conducted under the supervision of a physician with experience in recognizing and treating severe respiratory or systemic reactions and in centers with the necessary equipment for emergency resuscitation. Patients should be in stable condition and most guidelines recommend baseline forced expiratory volume in 1 second (FEV1) should be at least 60% to 70% predicted value. In patients with more compromised lung function who are undergoing inhalation challenge or OAC, initiation or escalation of oral corticosteroids should be considered. Intravenous line placement is recommended. Full informed consent should be obtained in all cases.[13,14]

Where lysine-aspirin is available, intranasal lysine-aspirin challenge can be performed in the outpatient setting.[13] In the case of OAC, accumulating experience and evidence supports performing OACs in the outpatient setting as long as the following criteria are met:

- Stable lung function and FEV1 $\geq$60% predicted
- Premedication with antileukotriene therapy and other appropriate asthma controller therapy
- Physician and nursing personnel experienced in OACs are present, and close monitoring is feasible[15]

Performing diagnostic challenges when the outcome is uncertain presents a potential challenge in clinical decision-making with regard to management of respiratory medications leading up to the challenge. The risks of withdrawing medications used for the treatment of asthma and/or CRSNP in hopes of not masking the signs and symptoms used to determine a positive test should be weighed against the benefits of continuing medications that may mask a positive result but create a safer outcome. Few studies have examined which medications have the potential to mask a positive reaction leading to a false-negative challenge. A study by White and colleagues[16] suggested that antileukotriene therapy, oral corticosteroids, inhaled corticosteroids, and long-acting beta-agonists appeared to reduce the risk of lower airway reactions in the oral challenge setting, but did not mask respiratory reactions. Other studies have suggested that antihistamines, leukotriene receptor antagonists, and 5-lipoxygenase inhibitors have the potential to mask a positive challenge.[17–21] However, because of studies that support enhanced safety of OACs in patients taking antileukotriene therapy and other controller therapy, current practice in the United States is to initiate or continue antileukotriene therapy, inhaled corticosteroids, and long-acting beta-agonists in preparation for OACs.[14–16,22] European guidelines, on the other hand, recommend conducting OACs after withdrawing antileukotriene therapy and long-acting beta-agonists.[13] **Table 2** lists the recommendations for medication withdrawal before NSAID challenges.

### Treatment of Positive Nonsteroidal Anti-Inflammatory Drug Challenges

Patients undergoing aspirin challenge should be warned that an NSAID-induced reaction is likely to occur that may require inhaled beta-agonists and even intramuscular epinephrine. Once a positive challenge has occurred, optimizing patient safety necessitates early, aggressive, and appropriate treatment of the reaction. **Table 3** lists treatment options for the most commonly observed reactions provoked by NSAID challenge. Anaphylaxis should be treated as outlined in anaphylaxis treatment guidelines.[23,24]

### Inhalation/Bronchial Challenge

First introduced in 1977, inhalation lysine-aspirin challenge is considered to be safer and less time-consuming than oral challenge but not as sensitive.[13,25] Systemic reactions to bronchial challenge have been reported.[26] In a protocol published in European guidelines, lysine-aspirin is administered as a graded challenge by nebulization beginning with a dose of 0.18 mg lysine-aspirin. Incrementally increasing doses are administered every 30 minutes, with FEV1 monitoring at baseline and every 10 minutes to a maximum cumulative dose of 181.98 mg.[13] The challenge is considered to be positive if FEV1 decreases by ≥20% as compared with baseline FEV1. The provoking dose (PD20) is then calculated and recorded. The challenge takes approximately 4 hours to complete. Because of the reduced sensitivity of inhalation challenge as compared with oral challenge, oral challenge is recommended following a negative inhalation challenge.[13]

### Intranasal Challenge

Intranasal challenge with lysine-aspirin or ketorolac has the advantage of being less likely to provoke a severe systemic or lower respiratory response, and is therefore

**Table 2**
**Medication withdrawal before diagnostic nonsteroidal anti-inflammatory drug challenge**

| Medication | European Guidelines | | US Guidelines |
|---|---|---|---|
| | Nasal | Bronchial/Oral | |
| Oral antihistamines | 24 h | 3 d | 48 h |
| Oral decongestants | 24 h | — | 48 h |
| Nasal cromolyn | 24 h | — | — |
| Leukotriene modifiers | ≥7 d | ≥7 d | — |
| Oral corticosteroids | 7 d | — | — |
| Nasal corticosteroids | 7 d | — | — |
| Inhaled corticosteroids | — | — | — |
| Long-acting beta-agonists | — | 24–48 h | — |
| Short-acting beta-agonists | — | 6–8 h | 6–8 h |
| Inhaled anticholinergics | — | 24 h | — |

*Data from* Nizankowska-Mogilnicka E, Bochenek G, Mastalerz L, et al. EAACI/GA2LEN guideline: aspirin provocation tests for diagnosis of aspirin hypersensitivity. Allergy 2007;62:1111–8; and Macy E, Bernstein JA, Castells MC, et al. Aspirin challenge and desensitization for aspirin-exacerbated respiratory disease: a practice paper. Ann Allergy Asthma Immunol 2007;98:172–4.

| Table 3 | |
|---|---|
| **Treatment of positive NSAID challenges** | |
| **Organ System** | **Medication Options** |
| Ocular | Oral antihistamines, ocular antihistamine/mast cell stabilizers |
| Nasal | Oral or nasal antihistamines, oral or nasal decongestants |
| Bronchial | Inhaled beta-agonists, inhaled anticholinergics |
| Laryngeal | Inhaled racemic epinephrine, intramuscular epinephrine |
| Cutaneous | Oral or intravenous antihistamines |
| Gastrointestinal | Oral or intravenous $H_2$-antihistamines, anti-dopaminergic anti-emetics |
| Vascular (hypotension) | Intramuscular epinephrine |

*Adapted from* Joint Task Force on Practice Parameters. Drug allergy: an updated practice parameter. Ann Allergy Asthma Immunol 2010;105:273.e41.

considered safer.[5,13] It should be noted, however, that systemic and lower airway reactions have been reported with intranasal ketorolac.[5] Intranasal lysine-aspirin challenge may be particularly useful in patients who lack clinically apparent asthma, who have severe or unstable lower airway disease, or who are at high risk of severe systemic or lower airway reactions.[13] Disadvantages include limitations of use in patients with severe nasal obstruction by massive, anteriorly extending polyps and reduced sensitivity. Four methods of assessment of response to nasal challenge include symptoms, acoustic rhinometry, active anterior rhinomanometry, and peak nasal inspiratory flow (PNIF).[13]

## Intranasal Lysine-Aspirin Challenge

After baseline assessment of symptoms and objective measurement of nasal patency and/or flow, intranasal saline is administered to evaluate for nonspecific nasal hyperreactivity. If there is a 20% change from baseline measurements after saline administration, the specificity of any attempt to provoke symptoms with lysine-aspirin would be very low and the challenge should not proceed further. Once nonspecific hyperreactivity is excluded, lysine-aspirin 80 µL (total aspirin dose of 16 mg) is instilled into each nostril and the patient's head is tilted back for 1 minute. Symptom and objective assessments are made every 10 minutes for 2 hours.

A positive response is defined as the development of nasal symptoms such as rhinorrhea, nasal congestion, or sneezing and a reduction in objective measurements of nasal patency and/or flow. For acoustic rhinometry, a positive test is defined as a ≥25% decrease from baseline in total nasal flow value at 12 cm. In the case of rhinomanometry or PNIF, a 40% decrease in flow as compared with baseline is required for a positive test. A study comparing the test performance characteristics of acoustic rhinometry and PNIF found acoustic rhinometry to have better sensitivity.[27] Because of the reduced sensitivity of intranasal challenge, a negative nasal challenge should be followed by OAC.[13]

## Intranasal Ketorolac and Modified Oral Aspirin Challenge

The barrier to topical airway provocation challenge in AERD presented by the lack of access to an aqueous NSAID (such as lysine-aspirin) in the United States was overcome by the development of intranasal ketorolac challenge by White and colleagues[4] in 2006. In this approach, ketorolac is applied to the nasal passage by metered dose nasal spray bottle, using incremental doses administered every 30 minutes with PNIF and spirometry measured before each dose (**Table 4**). A positive challenge is

**Table 4**
**Intranasal ketorolac and modified oral aspirin challenge dosing protocol**

| Day | Interval, min | Sprays, no. | Ketorolac Dose, mg | Ketorolac Cumulative Dose, mg | Aspirin Dose, mg | Aspirin Cumulative Dose, mg |
|---|---|---|---|---|---|---|
| 1 | — | 1 in 1 nostril | 1.26 | 1.26 | — | — |
|  | 30 | 1 in each nostril | 2.52 | 3.78 | — | — |
|  | 30 | 2 in each nostril | 5.04 | 8.82 | — | — |
|  | 30 | 3 in each nostril | 7.56 | 16.38 | — | — |
|  | 60 | — | — | — | 60 | 60 |
|  | 60 | — | — | — | 60 | 120 |
|  | 90 | (Observation) |  |  |  |  |
| 2 | — | — | — | — | 150 | 270 |
|  | 180 | — | — | — | 325 | 595 |
|  | 180 | (Observation) |  |  |  |  |

*Data from* Lee RU, White AA, Ding D, et al. Use of intranasal ketorolac and modified oral aspirin challenge for desensitization of aspirin-exacerbated respiratory disease. Ann Allergy Asthma Immunol 2010;105:130–5.

defined as development of symptoms of rhinitis, conjunctivitis, or bronchospasm with a decrease in PNIF of ≥20% and/or a decrease in FEV1 by ≥15% from baseline.[4,5] The dose provoking a positive reaction is repeated before progressing to the next dose.

The initial study of the use of intranasal ketorolac alone reported a sensitivity of 78% and a specificity of 64% for the diagnosis of AERD.[4] As a result, if the maximum dose of 3 sprays per nostril (total cumulative dose of ketorolac 16.38 mg) is reached without symptoms, a modified oral challenge is then performed. Preliminary results indicate that this is a safe technique, with a reduced risk of laryngospasm and gastrointestinal side effects. The intranasal ketorolac and modified OAC take an average of 1.9 days to complete.[5]

## Oral Aspirin Challenge

Oral aspirin challenge is considered to be the most conclusive way to confirm the diagnosis of AERD.[6,28] A number of protocols have been published for the purpose of OAC, and in most cases, these protocols are designed to convert a positive challenge into a completed desensitization in a single procedure. Four variations of published OAC protocols are presented in **Table 5**.

Baseline symptoms, FEV1, vital signs, and objective measurement of nasal flow/patency (where available) are assessed at baseline and at 30-minute to 60-minute intervals. Incremental doses are then given as dictated by the protocol until signs or symptoms of a reaction are observed. A positive oral challenge is defined by 1 or more of the following:

- Obvious signs and symptoms of respiratory reaction
  - Upper respiratory reaction (rhinorrhea, nasal congestion, sneezing, increased lacrimation)
  - Bronchospasm (coughing, wheezing, chest tightness, dyspnea)
  - Laryngospasm (stridor, dysphonia)
- Decrease in FEV1 by ≥15% or ≥20% (depending on the center)
- Decrease in nasal flow and/or patency (see section on Intranasal Lysine-Aspirin Challenge)

| Table 5 | | | |
|---|---|---|---|
| **Examples of published oral aspirin challenge protocols** | | | |
| Protocol Source | Dosing Interval, min | Doses, mg | Time to Complete, d |
| Scripps Clinic[15] | 180 | 20–40, 40–60, 60–100, 100–160, 160–325, 325 | ≥2 |
| EAACI Guidelines[13] | 90–120 | 10[a], 27, 44, 117, 312, 500 | ≥1 |
| Aspirin Desensitization Joint Task Force[14] | 90 | 20.25, 40.5, 81, 162.5, 325 | ≥1 |
| UTSW Medical Center[29] | 60 | 20[a], 40, 81, 120, 162, 325 | ≥1 |

*Abbreviations:* EAACI, European Academy of Allergy and Clinical Immunology; UTSW, University of Texas Southwestern.
[a] Lower starting dose is used if the patient has a history of a severe nonsteroidal anti-inflammatory drug–induced reaction.

Once AERD is confirmed with a positive reaction, the symptoms are treated aggressively (see **Table 3**). Once the symptoms have been controlled, most centers proceed with the process that leads to desensitization. This entails repeat administration of the provoking dose until no reaction is observed, then continuing with incremental doses as dictated by the protocol, repeating any dose that elicits further airway reactions before proceeding to the next dose.[13–15,28–30]

Starting doses and dosing intervals vary widely between published OAC protocols. The cited reason for this variation has to do with balancing time efficiency of the procedure with the risk of administering escalating doses prematurely. When a 3-hour dosing interval is used, the mean time elapsed from ingestion of the provoking dose of aspirin to onset of reaction was found to be 102 minutes and the mean provoking dose to be 68 mg, with most positive challenges occurring after doses of 45 to 100 mg aspirin.[31] Using a 60-minute dosing interval, Chen and colleagues[29] found the mean time to onset of symptoms to be 50 minutes and the mean provoking dose to be 157 mg. Whether the apparent shorter time to onset of symptoms and higher provoking dose in the latter study are due to attributing provocation of the reaction to the incorrect dose is not known. A theoretic concern of using a dosing interval of less than 90 minutes is that not enough observation time elapses to permit identification and treatment of a reaction in many patients before the next dose is given. Whether protocols with shorter dosing intervals are associated with more severe or difficult-to-treat OAC reactions has not been extensively evaluated. The preliminary report of 57 patients who underwent OAC and desensitization with the 60-minute dosing-interval protocol suggests this to be a safe approach in select patients.[29]

Most (90%–98%) positive oral challenges include a naso-ocular reaction, and 35% to 90% include a bronchial reaction.[29,31–33] Positive reactions also can include gastrointestinal symptoms (eg, abdominal pain, nausea, vomiting), cutaneous symptoms (eg, hives, itching, flushing), and laryngeal symptoms (eg, laryngeal edema or laryngospasm) with a frequency of 23%, 10%, and 8%, respectively, according to one analysis.[32] Hypotension also has been reported.[16]

Hope and colleagues[31] sought to identify risk factors that might predict a more severe bronchial reaction. Multivariate analysis suggested that the clinical predictors of moderate-to-severe bronchial reactions (defined as >20% decrease in FEV1 from pre-challenge baseline) include the following:

- Lack of prechallenge treatment with anti-leukotriene therapy
- Duration of symptoms of AERD ≤10 years

- Baseline FEV1 less than 80% predicted
- Prior emergency room visit for asthma exacerbation other than caused by NSAIDs, and lack of leukotriene modifier therapy at the time of challenge[31]

If 3 or more risk factors were present, the risk of a moderate-to-severe reaction was 43%.[31] On the other hand, the severity of the reaction reported by patients before OAC does not predict the severity of the reaction observed during OAC, with observed challenge reactions generally being milder.[32]

A negative challenge is defined as completing the challenge protocol until the maximum dose is reached (usually 325 mg aspirin) without any of the signs, symptoms, or objective measures of airway reaction defined previously. A patient with a high prechallenge probability of AERD, based on the available history, who then has a negative challenge presents a special challenge. The reported sensitivity of OAC of 90% indicates that the possibility of a false-negative challenge exists.[7,8,21] In addition, White and colleagues[21] reported a case series illustrating the clinical dilemma of "silent desensitization" in which patients with initial negative OACs were later confirmed to have AERD on repeat challenge. An approach to the patient with a high suspicion for AERD but a negative OAC involves either (1) repeat challenge when the patient is not receiving leukotriene therapy and oral steroids, perhaps including higher aspirin challenge doses, or (2) presumptive diagnosis of AERD and continuation of therapeutic doses of aspirin with assessment of symptom response at 6 months.[21]

### In Vitro Diagnostic Testing

Currently, the only reliable means of confirming the diagnosis of AERD is by provocation of respiratory or systemic hypersensitivity NSAID reactions. In vitro testing for AERD would offer a safer alternative to the current approach. A number of approaches are in development but none have proven to be reliable enough for clinical practice at this time. Examples include the cellular activation stimulation test, leukotriene release assay, basophil activation test, and the 15-hydroxyeicosatetranoic acid assay (ASPITest).[34–41]

### SUMMARY

In most cases, patients with clinical features of AERD would benefit from evaluation by a respiratory specialist with expertise in the diagnosis and management of AERD. Confirmation or exclusion of the diagnosis of AERD has important clinical implications. Most patients present with CRSNP, asthma, and a history of one or more episodes of respiratory or systemic reactions to ingestion of NSAIDs, whereas a smaller number of patients with CRSNP and/or asthma are uncertain as to their ability to tolerate NSAIDs. In the first case, diagnostic NSAID challenge is typically performed as part of aspirin desensitization, which confirms the diagnosis and permits long-term therapeutic use of aspirin. In the second case, NSAID challenge should be performed to either free the patient without AERD from the burden of lifelong NSAID avoidance or to confirm the presence of AERD and the management implications that this entails.

In experienced hands, these diagnostic challenges are relatively safe and increasingly performed in the outpatient setting. Where available, lysine-aspirin inhalational or intranasal challenges have an excellent safety record. OAC remains the gold standard for confirming the diagnosis of AERD. In the United States, the use of antileukotriene premedication and the development of intranasal ketorolac and modified OAC have contributed to enhanced safety of diagnostic challenges, as well.

Future work in the diagnosis of AERD will likely focus on continued efforts to optimize the safety and time efficiency of performing these diagnostic challenges in the outpatient setting. The hope of an accurate in vitro diagnostic test for AERD also remains.

## REFERENCES

1. Rajan JP, Wineinger NE, Stevenson DD, et al. Prevalence of aspirin-exacerbated respiratory disease among asthmatic patients: a meta-analysis of the literature. J Allergy Clin Immunol 2014;135:676–81.
2. Szczeklik A, Nizankowska E, Duplaga M, et al. Natural history of aspirin-induced asthma. Eur Respir J 2000;16:432–6.
3. Dursun AB, Woessner KA, Simon RA, et al. Predicting outcomes of oral aspirin challenges in patients with asthma, nasal polyps, and chronic sinusitis. Ann Allergy Asthma Immunol 2008;100:420–5.
4. White AA, Bigby TA, Stevenson DD. Intranasal ketorolac challenge for the diagnosis of aspirin exacerbated respiratory disease. Ann Allergy Asthma Immunol 2006;97:190–5.
5. Lee RU, White AA, Ding D, et al. Use of intranasal ketorolac and modified oral aspirin challenge for desensitization of aspirin-exacerbated respiratory disease. Ann Allergy Asthma Immunol 2010;105:130–5.
6. Bochenek G, Nizankowska-Mogilnicka E. Aspirin-exacerbated respiratory disease: clinical disease and diagnosis. Immunol Allergy Clin N Am 2013;33: 147–61.
7. Nizankowska E, Bestynska-Krypel A, Cmiel A, et al. Oral and bronchial provocation tests with aspirin for diagnosis of aspirin-induced asthma. Eur Respir J 2000; 15:863–9.
8. Dahlen B, Zetterstrom O. Comparison of bronchial and per oral provocation with aspirin in aspirin-sensitive asthmatics. Eur Respir J 1990;3:527–34.
9. Milewski M, Mastalerz L, Nizankowska E, et al. Nasal provocation test for diagnosis of aspirin-induced asthma. J Allergy Clin Immunol 1998;101:581–6.
10. Alonso-Llamazares A, Martinez-Cocera C, Dominiquez-Ortega J, et al. Nasal provocation test (NPT) with aspirin: a sensitive and safe method to diagnose aspirin-induced asthma (AIA). Allergy 2002;57:632–5.
11. Gonzalez-Perez R, Poza-Guedes P, Vives-Conesa R. The nose as a target organ in the diagnosis of severe aspirin-exacerbated respiratory disease. Am J Rhinol Allergy 2011;25:166–9.
12. Celikel S, Stevenson D, Erkorkmaz U, et al. Use of nasal inspiratory flow rates in the measurement of aspirin-induced respiratory reactions. Ann Allergy Asthma Immunol 2013;111:252–5.
13. Nizankowska-Mogilnicka E, Bochenek G, Mastalerz L, et al. EAACI/GA2LEN guideline: aspirin provocation tests for diagnosis of aspirin hypersensitivity. Allergy 2007;62:1111–8.
14. Macy E, Bernstein JA, Castells MC, et al. Aspirin challenge and desensitization for aspirin-exacerbated respiratory disease: a practice paper. Ann Allergy Asthma Immunol 2007;98:172–4.
15. White AA, Stevenson DD. Aspirin desensitization in AERD. Immunol Allergy Clin N Am 2013;33:211–22.
16. White AA, Stevenson DD, Simon RA. The blocking effect of essential controller medications during aspirin challenges in patients with aspirin-exacerbated respiratory disease. Ann Allergy Asthma Immunol 2005;95:330–5.

17. Szczeklik A, Serwonska M. Inhibition of idiosyncratic reactions to aspirin in asthmatic patients by clemastine. Thorax 1979;34:654–7.

18. Israel E, Fischer AR, Rosenberg MA, et al. The pivotal role of 5-lipoxygenase products in the reaction of aspirin-sensitive asthmatics to aspirin. Am Rev Respir Dis 1993;148:1447–51.

19. Stevenson DD, Simon RA, Mathison DA, et al. Montelukast is only partially effective in inhibiting aspirin responses in aspirin-sensitive asthmatics. Ann Allergy Asthma Immunol 2000;85:477–82.

20. White A, Ludington E, Mehra P, et al. Effect of leukotriene modifier drugs on the safety of oral aspirin challenges. Ann Allergy Asthma Immunol 2006;97:688–93.

21. White AA, Bosso JV, Stevenson DD. The clinical dilemma of "silent desensitization" in aspirin-exacerbated respiratory disease. Allergy Asthma Proc 2013;34: 378–82.

22. Berges-Gimeno MP, Simon RA, Stevenson DD. The effect of leukotriene-modifier drugs on aspirin-induced asthma and rhinitis reactions. Clin Exp Allergy 2002;32: 1491–6.

23. Simons FE, Ardusso LR, Dimov V, et al. World Allergy Organization Anaphylaxis Guidelines: 2013 update of the evidence base. Int Arch Allergy Immunol 2013; 162:193–204.

24. Dhami S, Panesar SS, Roberts G, et al. Management of anaphylaxis: a systematic review. Allergy 2014;69:168–75.

25. Bianco S, Robushi M, Patrigni G. Aspirin induced tolerance in aspirin-induced asthma detected by a new challenge test. J Med Sci 1977;5:129–30.

26. Makowska JS, Grzegorczyk J, Bienkiewicz B, et al. Systemic responses after bronchial aspirin challenge in sensitive patients with asthma. J Allergy Clin Immunol 2008;121:348–54.

27. Miller B, Mirakian R, Gane S, et al. Nasal lysine aspirin challenge in the diagnosis of aspirin-exacerbated respiratory disease. Clin Exp Allergy 2013;43:874–80.

28. Joint Task Force on Practice Parameters. Drug allergy: an updated practice parameter. Ann Allergy Asthma Immunol 2010;105:273.e1-e78.

29. Chen JR, Buchmiller BL, Khan DA. An hourly dose-escalation desensitization protocol for aspirin-exacerbated respiratory disease. J Allergy Clin Immunol Pract 2015;3:926–31.

30. Stevenson DD, Simon RA. Selection of patients for aspirin desensitization treatment. J Allergy Clin Immunol 2006;118:801–4.

31. Hope AP, Woessner KA, Simon RA, et al. Rational approach to aspirin dosing during oral challenges and desensitization of patients with aspirin-exacerbated respiratory disease. J Allergy Clin Immunol 2009;123:406–10.

32. Williams AN, Simon RA, Woessner KM, et al. The relationship between historical aspirin-induced asthma and severity of asthma induced during oral aspirin challenges. J Allergy Clin Immunol 2007;120:273–7.

33. Kowalski ML, Makowska JS, Blanca M, et al. Hypersensitivity to nonsteroidal anti-inflammatory drugs (NSAIDs)–classification, diagnosis and management: review of the EAACI/ENDA and GA2LEN/HANNA. Allergy 2011;66:818–29.

34. Bavbek S, Dursun AB, Birben E, et al. Cellular allergen stimulation test with acetylsalicylic acid-lysine is not a useful test to discriminate between asthmatic patients with and without acetylsalicylic acid sensitivity. Int Arch Allergy Immunol 2009;149:58–64.

35. Celik G, Bavbek S, Misirligil Z, et al. Release of cysteinyl leukotrienes with aspirin stimulation and the effect of prostaglandin E(2) on this release from peripheral

blood leucocytes in aspirin-induced asthmatic patients. Clin Exp Allergy 2001;31: 1615–22.

36. Pierzchalska M, Mastalerz L, Sanak M, et al. A moderate and unspecific release of cysteinyl leukotrienes by aspirin from peripheral blood leucocytes precludes its value for aspirin sensitivity testing in asthma. Clin Exp Allergy 2000;30:1785–91.

37. Sanz ML, Gamboa P, de Weck AL. A new combined test with flowcytometric basophil activation and determination of sulfidoleukotrienes is useful for in vitro diagnosis of hypersensitivity to aspirin and other non-steroidal anti-inflammatory drugs. Int Arch Allergy Immunol 2005;136:58–72.

38. Gamboa P, Sanz ML, Caballero MR, et al. The flow-cytometric determination of basophil activation induced by aspirin and other non-steroidal anti-inflammatory drugs (NSAIDs) is useful for in vitro diagnosis of the NSAID hypersensitivity syndrome. Clin Exp Allergy 2004;34:1448–57.

39. Sanz ML, Gamboa PM, Mayorga C. Basophil activation tests in the evaluation of immediate drug hypersensitivity. Curr Opin Allergy Clin Immunol 2009;9:298–304.

40. Kowalski ML, Ptasinska A, Jedrzejczak M, et al. Aspirin-triggered 15-HETE generation in peripheral blood leukocyte is specific and sensitive Aspirin-Sensitive Patients Identification Test (ASPITest). Allergy 2005;60:1139–45.

41. Jedrzejczak-Czechowicz M, Lewandowska-Polak A, Bienkiewicz B, et al. Involvement of 15-lipoxygenase and prosta-glandin EP receptors in aspirin-triggered 15-hydroxyeicosatetraenoic acid generation in aspirin-sensitive asthmatics. Clin Exp Allergy 2008;38:1108–16.

# Aspirin-Exacerbated Respiratory Disease as an Endotype of Chronic Rhinosinusitis

Whitney W. Stevens, MD, PhD[a], Robert P. Schleimer, PhD[a,b],*

## KEYWORDS

- Chronic rhinosinusitis • Chronic rhinosinusitis with nasal polyps • CRSwNP
- Aspirin-exacerbated respiratory disease • AERD • Samter disease • Samter triad

## KEY POINTS

- Clinically, patients with aspirin-exacerbated respiratory disease (AERD) can be distinguished from those with chronic rhinosinusitis with nasal polyps (CRSwNP) and asthma by the development of respiratory symptoms following the ingestion of a COX-1 inhibitor. However, clinical history alone may not always be sufficient to confirm the diagnosis of AERD.
- In the absence of COX-1 inhibitors, patients with AERD on average still have worse upper and lower respiratory tract disease than those patients with CRSwNP with or without asthma.
- Nasal polyps from patients with AERD and CRSwNP are both defined by a predominant type-2 inflammatory environment but there appears to be significantly increased levels of eosinophil and mast cell degranulation occurring in AERD.
- Mechanistically, AERD, unlike CRSwNP, is characterized by platelet activation as well as a dysregulation in arachidonic acid metabolism.

---

Disclosures: W.W. Stevens has no financial conflicts of interest. R.P. Schleimer has served as a consultant with several pharmaceutical companies with interest in CRS, including Astra-Zeneca, Genentech, GSK, Intersect ENT, Merck, Regeneron, and Sanofi. R.P. Schleimer is a founder, shareholder, and advisor for Allakos.
Funding: This work was supported by Chronic Rhinosinusitis Integrative Studies Program (U19-AI106683) and by the National Institutes of Health grants T32 AI083216, R37 HLO68546, RO1 HL0788860 and R01 AI104733.

[a] Division of Allergy-Immunology, Department of Medicine, Northwestern University Feinberg School of Medicine, 240 E. Huron St, Chicago, IL 60611, USA; [b] Department of Otolaryngology, Northwestern University Feinberg School of Medicine, 675 N St. Clair St Suite 15-200, Chicago, IL 60611, USA
* Corresponding author. Division of Allergy-Immunology, Northwestern University Feinberg School of Medicine, 240 East Huron Street, McGaw Room M-318, Chicago, IL 60611.
*E-mail address:* rpschleimer@northwestern.edu

Immunol Allergy Clin N Am 36 (2016) 669–680
http://dx.doi.org/10.1016/j.iac.2016.06.004 immunology.theclinics.com
0889-8561/16/$ – see front matter © 2016 Elsevier Inc. All rights reserved.

## INTRODUCTION

Chronic rhinosinusitis with nasal polyps (CRSwNP) and aspirin-exacerbated respiratory disease (AERD) are both conditions characterized by the presence of chronic sinonasal inflammation and nasal polyps. Numerous groups have labored to describe the clinical features of these diseases as well as investigate the underlying mechanisms that could be driving their overlapping but distinct pathophysiologic mechanisms. However, there are few head-to-head studies directly comparing the sinonasal inflammatory environment of CRSwNP with that of AERD. As a result, the relationship between CRSwNP and AERD remains incompletely defined.

## CLASSIFICATION

To further understand the relationship between CRSwNP and AERD, it is important to review the clinical criteria needed to make the diagnosis of each condition. Per the consensus guidelines, patients with CRSwNP must present with greater than 12 weeks of rhinorrhea, facial pressure or pain, nasal congestion, and/or a reduction in sense of smell.[1,2] Additionally, there must be objective evidence of nasal polyps and mucosal disease visualized on sinus computed tomography (CT) imaging or nasal endoscopy. CRSwNP can exist without medical comorbidities but more often is observed with other chronic conditions, such as asthma, hay fever, cystic fibrosis, or eosinophilic granulomatosis with polyangiitis.

The clinical diagnosis of AERD is based on evolving criteria. In 1922, Widal published the first study describing a patent with asthma, nasal polyps, and sensitivity to aspirin. Later, Samter and Beers[3] described a cohort of aspirin-sensitive patients of whom 85% had only respiratory symptoms and 51% had nasal polyps. In this report, it was noted "that every patient does not necessarily present with every potential component of the syndrome." Furthermore, later studies suggested that patients with AERD first developed upper respiratory tract symptoms that progressed to involve the lower respiratory tract and then last acquired the aspirin intolerance.[4] In 2001, the term "aspirin-exacerbated respiratory disease" was termed by Stevenson and colleagues[5] to emphasize that these patients had underlying respiratory disease that was worsened but not induced by aspirin. Additionally, over the course of time, it was also discovered that all medications that inhibit the cyclooxygenase-1 (COX-1) enzyme, not just aspirin, could elicit upper and lower respiratory tract symptoms in patients with AERD.

Given this history, it is not surprising that different terminologies are still used to define the same or related clinical phenotypes (eg, Samter disease, Samter triad, AERD, nonsteroidal anti-inflammatory disease–exacerbated respiratory disease, aspirin-intolerant asthma). However, even when the same terminology is used, there can be variations in the clinical features of the study cohort. For example, AERD has been investigated in patients with asthma and aspirin intolerance as well as in patients with asthma, aspirin intolerance, and CRSwNP. How the presence (or absence) of sinonasal inflammation might influence the overall disease pathology is not known. As a result, it is not clear whether these 2 groups are distinct subsets or rather part of a disease continuum. Unless otherwise specified, this review defines AERD as the presence of the triad of CRSwNP, asthma, and worsening of upper and lower respiratory tract symptoms following the ingestion of COX-1 inhibitors.

## EPIDEMIOLOGY

By definition, all patients with AERD have CRSwNP; however, not all patients with CRSwNP have AERD. It is estimated that only approximately 10% of patients with nasal polyps and approximately 9% of patients with chronic rhinosinusitis have AERD.[6] However, the true prevalence of AERD in the general population or among patients with both chronic rhinosinusitis and nasal polyps (CRSwNP) is still unknown. This is partly due to the lack of epidemiologic studies evaluating patients with CRSwNP in large primary care populations.

As an additional layer of complexity, both AERD and CRSwNP are associated with asthma. Nearly all patients with AERD and approximately 26% to 63% of patients with CRSwNP have asthma.[1,7,8] In contrast, only approximately 7% to 10% of patients with asthma have AERD but as many as 90% of patients with asthma may have radiographic evidence of sinonasal inflammation, with or without nasal polyps.[1,6,9,10] Interestingly, the prevalence of AERD can increase to approximately 15% among patients with severe asthma[6,9] and a significant association between severe asthma and enhanced sinonasal inflammation has been reported.[11] However, the true prevalence of AERD among patients with both CRSwNP and asthma is not known and, as a result, further investigation is needed.

## CLINICAL FEATURES

The respiratory reaction following ingestion of a COX-1 inhibitor is the most prominent and definitive clinical feature distinguishing patients with AERD from those with CRSwNP. In patients with AERD, this reaction is associated with distinct pathophysiological changes within the sinonasal mucosa. Consequently, most patients with AERD typically avoid taking COX-1 inhibitors of their own accord. This results in the presence of a population of patients with CRSwNP and asthma who have aspirin sensitivity that does not appear in their health records. Thus, diagnosis of AERD by examination of medical record charts can overlook a significant number of patients with AERD.

It has been reported that as many as 15% of asthmatic patients previously unaware of having a COX-1 inhibitor hypersensitivity had a positive reaction to aspirin during an oral challenge.[4] Additionally, in separate smaller studies of patients with both CRSwNP and asthma, 20% to 42% had positive aspirin challenges despite being previously unaware of any COX-1 hypersensitivity.[12,13] In contrast, it has been estimated that as many as 15% of patients with a clinical history consistent with the triad of AERD actually do not react to aspirin on clinical challenge and instead have only CRSwNP with asthma.[4,13,14] Taken together, these studies illustrate the limitations in distinguishing CRSwNP and AERD by clinical history alone and highlight the importance of confirming the diagnosis by oral aspirin challenge.

There are other less definitive clinical features that can help to distinguish between AERD and CRSwNP. Both CRSwNP and AERD develop in adulthood, with the average age of onset being approximately 42 and 34 years, respectively.[1,14] CRSwNP is more common in men whereas AERD is more common in women.[1,4,14] Interestingly, a more recent study examining patients who had undergone sinus surgery at a tertiary care hospital suggests that among patients with CRSwNP, women had more severe disease than men as determined by radiographic evidence of enhanced sinus inflammation, need for revision surgery, and use of oral corticosteroids at the time of surgery.[15] This is consistent with a large European cohort study that found that women with aspirin-induced asthma have more progressive upper and lower respiratory tract disease than men.[4]

Clinically, patients with CRSwNP or with AERD both present with symptoms of nasal congestion, rhinorrhea, sinus pressure/pain, and/or hyposmia. Patients with AERD were shown to subjectively report more severe sinus symptoms than patients with CRSwNP.[16] Additionally, patients with AERD typically have significantly worse endoscopic sinus scores as well as radiographic evidence of sinonasal inflammation compared with patients with CRSwNP.[16–18] Finally, patients with AERD have greater risk of symptom recurrence following surgery and are more likely to undergo revision surgeries sooner and more frequently than those without AERD.[19–21] The average number of revision surgeries in patients with AERD has been reported to range from 2.6 to 10.0.[4,14,21] In contrast, one study reported that patients with CRS on average underwent 1.8 total sinus surgeries but the number of revision surgeries in patients with CRSwNP specifically is not well established.[22]

With regard to lower respiratory tract disease, CRSwNP and AERD are both associated with asthma that is more severe than that in patients with asthma alone. Conversely, in patients with chronic rhinosinusitis undergoing surgery at a tertiary care facility, asthmatic patients had worse sinus scores than nonasthmatic patients.[23] Additionally, as mentioned previously, asthma severity increased with enhanced radiologic evidence of sinus severity.[11] In a separate study of 201 patients with AERD, 45% had uncontrolled asthma.[24] Additionally, Morales and colleagues[9] observed that patients with AERD had a 60% increase in risk of severe asthma and 80% increase in emergency room visits compared with patients with aspirin-tolerant asthma. Patients with AERD had lower mean bronchodilator forced expiratory volume in 1 second, more severe asthma by physician assessment, and higher intubation rates than patients without AERD.[25]

More recently, studies have begun to further define asthma characteristics, as there are variations within the population with regard to clinical features and overall disease severity. For example, the Severe Asthma Research Program performed a cluster analysis of more than 700 patients with persistent asthma and identified 5 distinct asthma subsets.[26] In particular, one of these cohorts (group 5) was characterized by having the most severe asthma, lowest baseline lung function, and frequent systemic corticosteroid use.[26] Additionally, almost half of these patients reported a history of sinus surgery,[26] again suggesting an association between asthma severity and chronic sinus disease. A similar cluster analysis was recently performed in a cohort of patients with AERD, albeit only approximately 81% reported a history of having nasal polyps. In this analysis, 4 distinct subgroups of AERD were defined predominantly based on levels of asthma severity ranging from mild to severe.[27] Interestingly, those patients with significant upper respiratory symptoms (group 1) had the highest levels of peripheral blood eosinophils and urinary leukotrienes among all the subsets examined.[27] It is thus clear that patients with nasal polyps and AERD have worse asthma than patients with asthma and no nasal polyps, and that patients with nasal polyps and asthma have worse nasal polyps than patients with nasal polyps and no asthma. These 2 diseases each appear to worsen the other.

A causal relationship between atopy and either CRSwNP or AERD is still not established and appears unlikely. It has been estimated that 51% to 86% of patients with CRSwNP[8,22] and 33% to 66% with AERD[4,14] are sensitized to at least one aeroallergen. However, it remains unclear whether allergic sensitization is associated with increased sinus disease severity.[8,22,23,28,29]

In summary, AERD, on average, is characterized by more severe upper airway disease than CRSwNP and more significant lower airway disease than asthma. As a result of the severity of their disease, patients with AERD place a disproportionate financial burden on the health care system compared with patients with either CRSwNP or asthma alone.[30] Given the heterogeneity in past AERD study populations, future investigations are needed to more extensively characterize patients with the clinical triad of AERD and directly compare them with patients with CRSwNP alone as well as with CRSwNP and asthma together. Such studies would also allow for a better understanding of the roles that gender, atopy, asthma, and intolerance to COX-1 inhibitors play in AERD versus CRSwNP.

## GENETICS

Because both CRSwNP and AERD develop in adulthood, neither a simple Mendelian pattern of inheritance nor a single genetic defect has been associated with either disease to date.[31,32] In support of this, cohort studies found that only 1% of American and 6% of European patients with AERD reported a family member also having AERD.[4,14] Additionally, there have been several studies evaluating whether various specific gene polymorphisms are linked to AERD, although not all patients with AERD evaluated in these analyses had CRSwNP (see previous discussion about definitions).[32–35] Taken together, the present data do not suggest a strong genetic component to CRSwNP or AERD but additional studies are clearly needed to definitively evaluate the role of genetic inheritance in CRSwNP and AERD.

As another means to search for potential gene expression differences between AERD and CRSwNP, Stankovic and colleagues[36] examined and compared transcriptional gene profiles of nasal polyps extracted from patients with CRSwNP, AERD, and healthy controls through a microarray analysis. Although specific gene signatures could distinguish AERD as well as CRSwNP nasal polyps from healthy sinonasal tissue, there were no significant differences in gene expression profiles between AERD and CRSwNP nasal polyps themselves. Interestingly, when compared with healthy controls, CRSwNP nasal polyps were specifically characterized by the upregulation of met proto-oncogene and protein phosphatase 1 regulatory subunit 9B as well as by the downregulation of prolactin-induced protein (PIP) and zinc alpha2-glycoprotein. In contrast, upregulation of periostin gene expression was most characteristic of AERD polyps compared with healthy controls.[36] The role these genes play in disease pathogenesis is uncertain but work from our laboratory has also confirmed a significant overlap between gene signature profiles of AERD and CRSwNP polyps (Stevens et al, unpublished data, 2016).

It is also possible that epigenetic changes and/or differential levels of various proteins or nonprotein inflammatory mediators could account for the clinical differences between the 2 conditions.[37] Alterations in gene expression could also be occurring in the bone marrow, in primary or secondary lymphoid tissues, or in other sites in AERD such that they are not detectable in nasal polyp tissue. Alternatively, unspecified external factors might be needed to induce the enhanced AERD phenotype observed in certain genetically susceptible patients with nasal polyps. As such, chronic viral infections, active smoking, and exposure to environmental tobacco smoke during childhood have all been hypothesized to play a role in the development of AERD.[38,39]

## DISEASE PATHOPHYSIOLOGY

Epithelial barrier dysfunction, exposures to pathogenic and nonpathogenic bacteria, and dysregulation of the host innate and adaptive immune responses are all thought to be important in CRSwNP pathophysiology. Unfortunately, less is known about the specific cellular and molecular mechanisms contributing to AERD pathogenesis in particular, especially at baseline when COX-1 inhibitors are not present. For example, the role of epithelial cells and the microbiome in AERD has not been as extensively characterized as it has in CRSwNP.[40–42] As a result, it is possible that specific functional and physical defects in sinonasal epithelial cells as well as alterations in the microbiome of the sinonasal cavity could distinguish AERD and CRSwNP clinical phenotypes. Clearly, further investigations are warranted.

## Host Immune Response

There has been an increasing focus on exploring how the host immune response could contribute to the chronic sinonasal inflammation seen in CRSwNP and AERD. One of the hallmarks of CRSwNP and AERD nasal polyps is an enhanced tissue eosinophilia compared with healthy sinonasal tissue.[43] Additionally, levels of the eosinophil granule protein, eosinophil cationic protein (ECP), were also significantly elevated in both subsets of nasal polyps compared with controls as well as in AERD nasal polyps compared with CRSwNP.[43–45] In contrast, recent studies found no significant difference in the number of eosinophils counted in hematoxylin and eosin–stained slides within nasal polyp sections from AERD and CRSwNP nasal polyps.[45,46] Taken together, these observations led to the hypothesis that eosinophils are more highly activated in AERD compared with CRSwNP, thus releasing their granule contents (causing more ECP to be detected in AERD) but in the process losing their ability to be detected by traditional histologic staining.

It should be noted that not all patients with CRSwNP have enhanced tissue eosinophilia. In particular, Asian patients either living in Asia or in the United States were found to have significantly fewer eosinophils in their nasal polyps when compared with patients with CRSwNP of European descent.[44,47] These observations would in turn suggest that Asian patients, given their relative paucity of tissue eosinophils, might be less likely to have AERD. This is supported by one small study from China that found the prevalence of AERD to be 0.57% among patients evaluated with CRSwNP,[48] which is must lower than the 9% to 10% estimated in a meta-analysis of patients predominantly of European descent.[6] Second-generation Asian individuals with CRSwNP in the United States also had less atopy and less comorbidity with asthma than individuals who were not Asian American. One interpretation of these findings is that the new generation of type 2 targeting biologicals may have reduced efficacy in patients of Asian descent.

In addition to eosinophils, CRSwNP nasal polyps are also traditionally characterized as having an increased number of innate type-2 lymphoid cells (ILC2), mast cells, basophils, and neutrophils when compared with healthy sinonasal tissue.[46,49–51] Walford and colleagues[50] reported an overall correlation between the number of eosinophils and ILC2s in nasal polyps but they did not specifically compare ILC2 numbers in AERD versus CRSwNP nasal polyps. Similar to eosinophils, mast cell numbers did not significantly differ between CRSwNP and AERD nasal polyps.[41,52] However, mast cells are a major source of prostaglandin D2 ($PGD_2$) and this inflammatory mediator has been shown to be significantly elevated in AERD compared with patients with CRSwNP, especially after aspirin challenge.[52,53] Finally, basophil numbers were significantly reduced in AERD versus CRSwNP nasal polyps.[46] It remains unclear exactly how eosinophils, basophils, mast cells, and ILC2s each contribute to sinonasal inflammation and the clinical symptoms of either CRSwNP or AERD. Furthermore, given the elevated levels of $PGD_2$ and ECP despite a lack of significant elevation in number of mast cells or eosinophils, it is tempting to speculate that these innate immune cells are more activated in AERD than CRSwNP. However, additional studies are needed to further evaluate this hypothesis.

Even less is known regarding adaptive immune cells in AERD. T cells are elevated in nasal polyps of patients with CRSwNP compared with healthy controls.[43,54] Additionally, B cells and plasma cells are also elevated in CRSwNP nasal polyps and thought to be locally activated within this tissue to produce increased amounts of immunoglobulin (Ig)G, IgA, IgM, and IgE.[43,55–57] Some of the antibodies found in CRSwNP nasal polyps are against self-proteins (eg, nuclear antigens and cytokines) but it is unclear if similar levels of autoantibodies exist in patients with AERD.[58,59]

It has been estimated that as many as 64% of patients with CRSwNP and 87% of patients with AERD are colonized with *Staphylococcus aureus* with a subset of these patients producing IgE against staphylococcal superantigens.[60] Some studies report significantly increased levels of IgE to staphylococcal superantigens in AERD nasal polyps compared with CRSwNP,[61,62] whereas a more recent study found no difference.[63] Taken together, additional studies are needed to further define the relationship between IgE to staphylococcal superantigens in AERD and CRSwNP nasal polyps. However, these specific antibodies may still contribute by an unknown mechanism to the chronic sinonasal inflammation observed in both diseases. In addition, *S aureus* enterotoxins can activate large numbers of T cells, and there is a body of literature suggesting that T-cell activation mediated by these toxins plays a role in CRSwNP.[64–66]

### Arachidonic Acid Metabolites

AERD is classically characterized by a systemic dysregulation in arachidonic acid metabolism, but a full description of this pathway is beyond the scope of this review. There have been some studies that have specifically focused on examination of prostaglandin and leukotriene mediators in the sinonasal tissue of patients with AERD compared with patients with CRSwNP. For example, levels of prostaglandin E2 ($PGE_2$), along with its receptor $EP_2$, are decreased in AERD versus CRSwNP nasal polyps.[67–70] Given the anti-inflammatory properties of $PGE_2$, its reduction in AERD could in turn contribute to the enhanced sinonasal inflammation observed.

Laidlaw and colleagues[71] recently reported that the number of platelet-adherent leukocytes was significantly increased in AERD compared with CRSwNP nasal polyps. Furthermore, these platelets could convert leukocyte-derived leukotriene (LT) $A_4$ into $LTC_4$ and thus contribute to the elevated levels of cysteinyl leukotrienes that are classically seen in AERD nasal polyps compared with CRSwNP or healthy controls.[67,71] Furthermore, the cysteinyl leukotriene receptor, CysLT1, is also elevated in AERD versus CRSwNP.[68,72,73] Interestingly, in CRSwNP, cysteinyl leukotrienes ($LTC_4$, $LTD_4$, and $LTE_4$) were also significantly elevated in sinonasal tissue when compared with healthy mucosae.[69,74] How these mediators all contribute to different clinical phenotypes in AERD versus CRSwNP is still not entirely understood.

### Other Inflammatory Mediators

In addition to arachidonic acid metabolites, there have been numerous studies characterizing the baseline inflammatory milieu of nasal polyps from patients with CRSwNP and patients with AERD. Given the association with type-2 innate immune cells (eg, mast cells, eosinophils, and basophils), it is not surprising that there are elevations in levels of traditional type-2 inflammatory mediators in AERD and also in CRSwNP nasal polyps when compared with healthy sinonasal tissue (eg, IL-5, IL-4, IL-13, Eotaxin-1, Eotaxin-2).[43–45,48,75,76]

However, when directly comparing AERD nasal polyps with CRSwNP nasal polyps, there have been conflicting results. Some reports suggest that protein levels of IL-5 and the type-1 cytokine, interferon (IFN)γ, are elevated in AERD compared with CRSwNP polyps.[67,77] More recently, a separate study evaluated the expression of 19 different inflammatory mediators in AERD and CRSwNP polyps. Surprisingly, there were no differences in levels of type-2 cytokines (IL-4, IL-5, IL-13, Eotaxin-1, Eotaxin-2, and MCP-4) or type-1 cytokines (IL-6, IFNγ) between these diseases,[45] although levels of GM-CSF and MCP-1 were significantly elevated in AERD nasal polyps.[45] It is unclear why there are discrepancies among studies but possible explanations could include differences in the tissues collected, techniques used to measure protein levels, the use of corticosteroids or other drugs within the study populations, and so forth.

In summary, it appears that both CRSwNP and AERD are characterized by a type-2 inflammatory milieu with increased levels of both type-2 cytokines and eosinophils when compared with healthy sinonasal tissue but not necessarily when compared with each other. There is a marked increase in levels of certain mediators released by activated innate immune cells (eg, ECP and $PGD_2$) in AERD compared with CRSwNP. Although the underlying mechanisms that contribute to the increase in inflammatory cell degranulation products is unknown, it is worth exploring whether the abnormalities in arachidonic acid metabolism or other factors mediate the exaggerated activation of these cells in AERD.

## SUMMARY

CRSwNP and AERD are both important clinical diseases associated with increased socioeconomic burden and decreased quality of life. The most prominent clinical feature distinguishing patients with AERD from those with CRSwNP remains the development of an upper or lower respiratory tract reaction following the ingestion of a COX-1 inhibitor. However, even in the absence of COX-1 inhibitors, there are other clinical and pathophysiological differences observed between patients with AERD and patients with CRSwNP. Those with AERD on average have worse upper respiratory disease with increased sinonasal symptoms, mucosal inflammation, and requirements for revision sinus surgery when compared with patients with CRSwNP. Although no single genetic factor has been identified in either CRSwNP or AERD pathogenesis to date, studies characterizing differences in the underlying cellular and molecular mechanisms that could account for the observed clinical variations are progressing. Both AERD and CRSwNP nasal polyps are now known to be characterized by a type-2 inflammatory environment, but there appear to be significantly increased levels of eosinophil and mast cell degranulation occurring in AERD sinonasal tissue. In addition, AERD, unlike CRSwNP, is also characterized by the systemic dysregulation of arachidonic acid metabolism and activation of platelet function. The underlying mechanisms that contribute to these observations are still not fully known and additional studies are needed to further define both CRSwNP and AERD pathogenesis.

## REFERENCES

1. Fokkens WJ, Lund VJ, Mullol J, et al. European position paper on rhinosinusitis and nasal polyps 2012. Rhinol Suppl 2012;(23). 3 p preceding table of contents, 1-298.
2. Peters AT, Spector S, Hsu J, et al. Diagnosis and management of rhinosinusitis: a practice parameter update. Ann Allergy Asthma Immunol 2014;113:347–85.
3. Samter M, Beers RF Jr. Intolerance to aspirin. Clinical studies and consideration of its pathogenesis. Ann Intern Med 1968;68:975–83.
4. Szczeklik A, Nizankowska E, Duplaga M. Natural history of aspirin-induced asthma. AIANE Investigators. European Network on Aspirin-Induced Asthma. Eur Respir J 2000;16:432–6.
5. Stevenson DD, Sanchez-Borges M, Szczeklik A. Classification of allergic and pseudoallergic reactions to drugs that inhibit cyclooxygenase enzymes. Ann Allergy Asthma Immunol 2001;87:177–80.

6. Rajan JP, Wineinger NE, Stevenson DD, et al. Prevalence of aspirin-exacerbated respiratory disease among asthmatic patients: a meta-analysis of the literature. J Allergy Clin Immunol 2015;135:676–81.e1.

7. Promsopa C, Kansara S, Citardi MJ, et al. Prevalence of confirmed asthma varies in chronic rhinosinusitis subtypes. Int Forum Allergy Rhinol 2016;6(4):373–7.

8. Tan BK, Zirkle W, Chandra RK, et al. Atopic profile of patients failing medical therapy for chronic rhinosinusitis. Int Forum Allergy Rhinol 2011;1:88–94.

9. Morales DR, Guthrie B, Lipworth BJ, et al. NSAID-exacerbated respiratory disease: a meta-analysis evaluating prevalence, mean provocative dose of aspirin and increased asthma morbidity. Allergy 2015;70:828–35.

10. Joe SA, Thakkar K. Chronic rhinosinusitis and asthma. Otolaryngol Clin North Am 2008;41:297–309, vi.

11. Lin DC, Chandra RK, Tan BK, et al. Association between severity of asthma and degree of chronic rhinosinusitis. Am J Rhinol Allergy 2011;25:205–8.

12. Delaney JC. The diagnosis of aspirin idiosyncrasy by analgesic challenge. Clin Allergy 1976;6:177–81.

13. Dursun AB, Woessner KA, Simon RA, et al. Predicting outcomes of oral aspirin challenges in patients with asthma, nasal polyps, and chronic sinusitis. Ann Allergy Asthma Immunol 2008;100:420–5.

14. Berges-Gimeno MP, Simon RA, Stevenson DD. The natural history and clinical characteristics of aspirin-exacerbated respiratory disease. Ann Allergy Asthma Immunol 2002;89:474–8.

15. Stevens WW, Peters AT, Suh L, et al. A retrospective, cross-sectional study reveals that women with CRSwNP have more severe disease than men. Immun Inflamm Dis 2015;3:14–22.

16. Jang DW, Comer BT, Lachanas VA, et al. Aspirin sensitivity does not compromise quality-of-life outcomes in patients with Samter's triad. Laryngoscope 2014;124: 34–7.

17. Awad OG, Lee JH, Fasano MB, et al. Sinonasal outcomes after endoscopic sinus surgery in asthmatic patients with nasal polyps: a difference between aspirin-tolerant and aspirin-induced asthma? Laryngoscope 2008;118:1282–6.

18. Robinson JL, Griest S, James KE, et al. Impact of aspirin intolerance on outcomes of sinus surgery. Laryngoscope 2007;117:825–30.

19. Young J, Frenkiel S, Tewfik MA, et al. Long-term outcome analysis of endoscopic sinus surgery for chronic sinusitis. Am J Rhinol 2007;21:743–7.

20. Yip J, Yao CM, Lee JM. State of the art: a systematic review of the surgical management of aspirin exacerbated respiratory disease. Am J Rhinol Allergy 2014; 28:493–501.

21. Kim JE, Kountakis SE. The prevalence of Samter's triad in patients undergoing functional endoscopic sinus surgery. Ear Nose Throat J 2007;86:396–9.

22. Batra PS, Tong L, Citardi MJ. Analysis of comorbidities and objective parameters in refractory chronic rhinosinusitis. Laryngoscope 2013;123(Suppl 7):S1–11.

23. Pearlman AN, Chandra RK, Chang D, et al. Relationships between severity of chronic rhinosinusitis and nasal polyposis, asthma, and atopy. Am J Rhinol Allergy 2009;23:145–8.

24. Bochenek G, Szafraniec K, Kuschill-Dziurda J, et al. Factors associated with asthma control in patients with aspirin-exacerbated respiratory disease. Respir Med 2015;109:588–95.

25. Lee JH, Haselkorn T, Borish L, et al. Risk factors associated with persistent airflow limitation in severe or difficult-to-treat asthma: insights from the TENOR study. Chest 2007;132:1882–9.

26. Moore WC, Meyers DA, Wenzel SE, et al. Identification of asthma phenotypes using cluster analysis in the Severe Asthma Research Program. Am J Respir Crit Care Med 2010;181:315–23.
27. Bochenek G, Kuschill-Dziurda J, Szafraniec K, et al. Certain subphenotypes of aspirin-exacerbated respiratory disease distinguished by latent class analysis. J Allergy Clin Immunol 2014;133:98–103.e1-6.
28. Robinson S, Douglas R, Wormald PJ. The relationship between atopy and chronic rhinosinusitis. Am J Rhinol 2006;20:625–8.
29. Ramadan HH, Fornelli R, Ortiz AO, et al. Correlation of allergy and severity of sinus disease. Am J Rhinol 1999;13:345–7.
30. Chang JE, White A, Simon RA, et al. Aspirin-exacerbated respiratory disease: burden of disease. Allergy Asthma Proc 2012;33:117–21.
31. Hsu J, Avila PC, Kern RC, et al. Genetics of chronic rhinosinusitis: state of the field and directions forward. J Allergy Clin Immunol 2013;131:977–93, 93.e1-5.
32. Park SM, Park JS, Park HS, et al. Unraveling the genetic basis of aspirin hypersensitivity in asthma beyond arachidonate pathways. Allergy Asthma Immunol Res 2013;5:258–76.
33. Kurosawa M, Yukawa T, Hozawa S, et al. Recent advance in investigation of gene polymorphisms in Japanese patients with aspirin-exacerbated respiratory disease. Allergol Immunopathol (Madr) 2015;43:92–100.
34. Kim SH, Choi H, Yoon MG, et al. Dipeptidyl-peptidase 10 as a genetic biomarker for the aspirin-exacerbated respiratory disease phenotype. Ann Allergy Asthma Immunol 2015;114:208–13.
35. Chang HS, Park JS, Shin HR, et al. Association analysis of FABP1 gene polymorphisms with aspirin-exacerbated respiratory disease in asthma. Exp Lung Res 2014;40:485–94.
36. Stankovic KM, Goldsztein H, Reh DD, et al. Gene expression profiling of nasal polyps associated with chronic sinusitis and aspirin-sensitive asthma. Laryngoscope 2008;118:881–9.
37. Cheong HS, Park SM, Kim MO, et al. Genome-wide methylation profile of nasal polyps: relation to aspirin hypersensitivity in asthmatics. Allergy 2011;66:637–44.
38. Szczeklik A. Aspirin-induced asthma as a viral disease. Clin Allergy 1988;18:15–20.
39. Chang JE, Ding D, Martin-Lazaro J, et al. Smoking, environmental tobacco smoke, and aspirin-exacerbated respiratory disease. Ann Allergy Asthma Immunol 2012;108:14–9.
40. Mahdavinia M, Keshavarzian A, Tobin MC, et al. A comprehensive review of the nasal microbiome in chronic rhinosinusitis (CRS). Clin Exp Allergy 2016;46:21–41.
41. Stevens WW, Lee RJ, Schleimer RP, et al. Chronic rhinosinusitis pathogenesis. J Allergy Clin Immunol 2015;136:1442–53.
42. Lou H, Meng Y, Piao Y, et al. Cellular phenotyping of chronic rhinosinusitis with nasal polyps. Rhinology 2016;54(2):150–9.
43. Van Zele T, Claeys S, Gevaert P, et al. Differentiation of chronic sinus diseases by measurement of inflammatory mediators. Allergy 2006;61:1280–9.
44. Zhang N, Van Zele T, Perez-Novo C, et al. Different types of T-effector cells orchestrate mucosal inflammation in chronic sinus disease. J Allergy Clin Immunol 2008;122:961–8.
45. Stevens WW, Ocampo CJ, Berdnikovs S, et al. Cytokines in chronic rhinosinusitis: role in eosinophilia and aspirin exacerbated respiratory disease. Am J Respir Crit Care Med 2015;192(6):682–94.

46. Mahdavinia M, Carter RG, Ocampo CJ, et al. Basophils are elevated in nasal polyps of patients with chronic rhinosinusitis without aspirin sensitivity. J Allergy Clin Immunol 2014;133:1759–63.

47. Mahdavinia M, Suh LA, Carter RG, et al. Increased noneosinophilic nasal polyps in chronic rhinosinusitis in US second-generation Asians suggest genetic regulation of eosinophilia. J Allergy Clin Immunol 2015;135:576–9.

48. Fan Y, Feng S, Xia W, et al. Aspirin-exacerbated respiratory disease in China: a cohort investigation and literature review. Am J Rhinol Allergy 2012;26:e20–2.

49. Ho J, Bailey M, Zaunders J, et al. Group 2 innate lymphoid cells (ILC2s) are increased in chronic rhinosinusitis with nasal polyps or eosinophilia. Clin Exp Allergy 2015;45:394–403.

50. Walford HH, Lund SJ, Baum RE, et al. Increased ILC2s in the eosinophilic nasal polyp endotype are associated with corticosteroid responsiveness. Clin Immunol 2014;155:126–35.

51. Takabayashi T, Kato A, Peters AT, et al. Glandular mast cells with distinct phenotype are highly elevated in chronic rhinosinusitis with nasal polyps. J Allergy Clin Immunol 2012;130:410–20.e5.

52. Buchheit KM, Cahill KN, Katz HR, et al. Thymic stromal lymphopoietin controls prostaglandin D generation in patients with aspirin-exacerbated respiratory disease. J Allergy Clin Immunol 2015;137(5):1566–76.e5.

53. Cahill KN, Bensko JC, Boyce JA, et al. Prostaglandin D(2): a dominant mediator of aspirin-exacerbated respiratory disease. J Allergy Clin Immunol 2015;135: 245–52.

54. Derycke L, Eyerich S, Van Crombruggen K, et al. Mixed T helper cell signatures in chronic rhinosinusitis with and without polyps. PLoS One 2014;9:e97581.

55. Van Zele T, Gevaert P, Holtappels G, et al. Local immunoglobulin production in nasal polyposis is modulated by superantigens. Clin Exp Allergy 2007;37: 1840–7.

56. Hulse KE, Norton JE, Suh L, et al. Chronic rhinosinusitis with nasal polyps is characterized by B-cell inflammation and EBV-induced protein 2 expression. J Allergy Clin Immunol 2013;131:1075–83, 83.e1–7.

57. Kato A, Peters A, Suh L, et al. Evidence of a role for B cell-activating factor of the TNF family in the pathogenesis of chronic rhinosinusitis with nasal polyps. J Allergy Clin Immunol 2008;121:1385–92, 92.e1–2.

58. Tan BK, Li QZ, Suh L, et al. Evidence for intranasal antinuclear autoantibodies in patients with chronic rhinosinusitis with nasal polyps. J Allergy Clin Immunol 2011;128:1198–206.e1.

59. Tsybikov NN, Egorova EV, Kuznik BI, et al. Anticytokine autoantibodies in chronic rhinosinusitis. Allergy Asthma Proc 2015;36:473–80.

60. Van Zele T, Gevaert P, Watelet JB, et al. Staphylococcus aureus colonization and IgE antibody formation to enterotoxins is increased in nasal polyposis. J Allergy Clin Immunol 2004;114:981–3.

61. Perez-Novo CA, Kowalski ML, Kuna P, et al. Aspirin sensitivity and IgE antibodies to Staphylococcus aureus enterotoxins in nasal polyposis: studies on the relationship. Int Arch Allergy Immunol 2004;133:255–60.

62. Suh YJ, Yoon SH, Sampson AP, et al. Specific immunoglobulin E for staphylococcal enterotoxins in nasal polyps from patients with aspirin-intolerant asthma. Clin Exp Allergy 2004;34:1270–5.

63. Yoo HS, Shin YS, Liu JN, et al. Clinical significance of immunoglobulin E responses to staphylococcal superantigens in patients with aspirin-exacerbated respiratory disease. Int Arch Allergy Immunol 2013;162:340–5.

64. Conley DB, Tripathi A, Seiberling KA, et al. Superantigens and chronic rhinosinusitis: skewing of T-cell receptor V beta-distributions in polyp-derived CD4+ and CD8+ T cells. Am J Rhinol 2006;20:534–9.
65. Huvenne W, Hellings PW, Bachert C. Role of staphylococcal superantigens in airway disease. Int Arch Allergy Immunol 2013;161:304–14.
66. Bachert C, Zhang N, Patou J, et al. Role of staphylococcal superantigens in upper airway disease. Curr Opin Allergy Clin Immunol 2008;8:34–8.
67. Perez-Novo CA, Watelet JB, Claeys C, et al. Prostaglandin, leukotriene, and lipoxin balance in chronic rhinosinusitis with and without nasal polyposis. J Allergy Clin Immunol 2005;115:1189–96.
68. Adamusiak AM, Stasikowska-Kanicka O, Lewandowska-Polak A, et al. Expression of arachidonate metabolism enzymes and receptors in nasal polyps of aspirin-hypersensitive asthmatics. Int Arch Allergy Immunol 2012;157:354–62.
69. Yoshimura T, Yoshikawa M, Otori N, et al. Correlation between the prostaglandin D(2)/E(2) ratio in nasal polyps and the recalcitrant pathophysiology of chronic rhinosinusitis associated with bronchial asthma. Allergol Int 2008;57:429–36.
70. Machado-Carvalho L, Torres R, Perez-Gonzalez M, et al. Altered expression and signalling of EP2 receptor in nasal polyps of AERD patients: role in inflammation and remodelling. Rhinology 2016. [Epub ahead of print].
71. Laidlaw TM, Kidder MS, Bhattacharyya N, et al. Cysteinyl leukotriene overproduction in aspirin-exacerbated respiratory disease is driven by platelet-adherent leukocytes. Blood 2012;119:3790–8.
72. Sousa AR, Parikh A, Scadding G, et al. Leukotriene-receptor expression on nasal mucosal inflammatory cells in aspirin-sensitive rhinosinusitis. N Engl J Med 2002; 347:1493–9.
73. Corrigan C, Mallett K, Ying S, et al. Expression of the cysteinyl leukotriene receptors cysLT(1) and cysLT(2) in aspirin-sensitive and aspirin-tolerant chronic rhinosinusitis. J Allergy Clin Immunol 2005;115:316–22.
74. Perez-Novo CA, Claeys C, Van Cauwenberge P, et al. Expression of eicosanoid receptors subtypes and eosinophilic inflammation: implication on chronic rhinosinusitis. Respir Res 2006;7:75.
75. Van Bruaene N, Perez-Novo CA, Basinski TM, et al. T-cell regulation in chronic paranasal sinus disease. J Allergy Clin Immunol 2008;121:1435–41, 1441.e1–3.
76. Steinke JW, Payne SC, Borish L. Interleukin-4 in the generation of the AERD phenotype: implications for molecular mechanisms driving therapeutic benefit of aspirin desensitization. J Allergy (Cairo) 2012;2012:182090.
77. Steinke JW, Liu L, Huyett P, et al. Prominent role of IFN-gamma in patients with aspirin-exacerbated respiratory disease. J Allergy Clin Immunol 2013;132: 856–65.e1-3.

# Pathogenesis of Aspirin-Induced Reactions in Aspirin-Exacerbated Respiratory Disease

Katherine N. Cahill, MD, Tanya M. Laidlaw, MD*

## KEYWORDS

- Aspirin-exacerbated respiratory disease • Pathogenesis • Cysteinyl leukotrienes
- Prostaglandins • Mast cell • Platelet-leukocyte aggregates

## KEY POINTS

- Aspirin-induced reactions in aspirin-exacerbated respiratory disease (AERD) result from the inhibition of COX-1 and cause a spectrum of reaction symptoms that range from localized respiratory symptoms to systemic symptoms involving the gastrointestinal tract and skin.
- The route of aspirin exposure and premedication with leukotriene modifying drugs (LTMDs) (ie, montelukast, zafirlukast or zileuton) influence the severity of aspirin-induced reactions. Intranasal desensitization protocols and the use of LTMDs allow for decreased bronchospasm and lowered rates of extrarespiratory symptoms.
- The release of tryptase, cysteinyl leukotrienes, histamine, and prostaglandin $D_2$ supports a central role for the mast cell in aspirin-induced reactions.
- Platelet-leukocyte aggregates are increased in AERD and are hypothesized to contribute to the overproduction of cysteinyl leukotrienes.
- Future studies of therapeutics that target mast cells, eosinophils, platelets, and inflammatory lipid and innate type 2 immune mediators in carefully phenotyped subjects are the key to improving our understanding of the classic aspirin-induced reactions in AERD.

## INTRODUCTION

Aspirin-exacerbated respiratory disease (AERD) encompasses 2 distinct disease phases: the chronic baseline inflammation of the upper and lower respiratory tract characterized by nasal polyposis and asthma and the acute hypersensitivity reactions triggered by inhibitors of cyclooxygenase (COX)-1. As Drs Stevenson and Szczeklik[1]

---

Disclosures: The authors have no relevant disclosures to report.
Division of Rheumatology, Immunology and Allergy, Brigham and Women's Hospital, Harvard Medical School, 1 Jimmy Fund Way, Smith Building, Room 638, Boston, MA 02115, USA
* Corresponding author. Brigham and Women's Hospital, 1 Jimmy Fund Way, Smith Building, Room 626B, Boston, MA 02115.
E-mail address: tlaidlaw@partners.org

Immunol Allergy Clin N Am 36 (2016) 681–691
http://dx.doi.org/10.1016/j.iac.2016.06.005
0889-8561/16/$ – see front matter © 2016 Elsevier Inc. All rights reserved.
immunology.theclinics.com

nicely observed, "exposure to aspirin [or other COX-1 inhibitors] does not initiate or even perpetuate the underlying respiratory inflammatory disease"[1]; yet the acutely exaggerated pathophysiology observed in the setting of an aspirin-induced respiratory reaction not only serves as the diagnostic gold standard but also offers insight into the cellular and biochemical derangements that underlie AERD. Our current understanding of the pathogenesis of aspirin reactions in AERD comes from studies of aspirin challenges performed in carefully phenotyped subjects. Our future progress in this disease lies in interventional trials of targeted therapeutics in the same carefully phenotyped populations.

## CLINICAL FEATURES OF REACTIONS

The consistent clinical features of aspirin-induced reactions have greatly informed our current understanding of the pathophysiology of AERD. Classically, exposure to aspirin elicits upper and/or lower respiratory symptoms within 30 to 180 minutes in patients with AERD. In addition to aspirin, these respiratory reactions are triggered by any inhibitor of COX-1 (eg, ibuprofen, naproxen, ketorolac) and can even be triggered by high doses of acetaminophen ($\geq$650 mg), which has mild COX-1 inhibitor properties,[2] but not by selective COX-2 inhibitors.[3,4] These reactions represent hypersensitivity reactions, which are not immunoglobulin (Ig) E–dependent and, therefore, are not formally classified as allergic.

In North America there are 2 well-validated and most often clinically applied aspirin challenge protocols,[5,6] involving oral aspirin and/or intranasal instillation of ketorolac, with a third protocol in Europe[7] that uses intranasal lysine aspirin. In addition to respiratory symptoms, a subset of patients with AERD also develops extrarespiratory or systemic symptoms involving the skin and gastrointestinal tract following exposure to a COX-1 inhibitor.[6,8] The route of aspirin challenge and the premedication regimen selected are the key predictors of both respiratory symptom severity and rates of extrarespiratory symptoms. In a study of 677 patients undergoing an oral aspirin challenge protocol, 38.6% of patients who were not on a leukotriene-modifying drug (LTMD) (n = 417) had a decrease in forced expiratory volume in the first second of expiration ($FEV_1$) of greater than 20%.[9] Whereas, of the 260 patients on an LTMD (ie, montelukast, zafirlukast, or zileuton), only 17.7% of patients had a decrease in $FEV_1$ of greater than 20%.[9] No benefit was seen with systemic steroids in this population; no comment was made on the change in rates of extrarespiratory symptoms, which were observed in less than 20% of the total study population. Further work has shown that on occasion LTMDs can completely prevent reaction symptoms during an oral aspirin challenge.[10] These effects of LTMDs support our current understanding of the cysteinyl leukotriene (cysLT) derangements in AERD and are covered in greater detail later.

Changing the route of aspirin exposure from oral to intranasal decreases the severity of the respiratory and extrarespiratory symptoms observed during the aspirin challenge. Because the soluble form of aspirin, lysine aspirin, is not available in the United States, the standard intranasal protocol uses intranasal ketorolac over 4 doses before completing the protocol with oral aspirin at 60 mg, 100 mg, 160 mg, and 325 mg.[11] A study of 100 patients desensitized using this intranasal ketorolac protocol demonstrated that it can be a safer way of inducing desensitization when compared with 100 patients desensitized using only oral aspirin. Intranasal ketorolac decreased the mean decrease in $FEV_1$ (average decrease of 13.4% in oral challenge vs 8.5% in intranasal) and decreased the percentage of patients who developed extrapulmonary reactions (23% with intranasal ketorolac vs 45% with oral challenge), particularly laryngospasm (7% vs 19%; $P = .02$) and gastrointestinal reactions (12% vs 33%; $P = .001$).[6] Thus, intranasal protocols increase the safety of desensitizations while accomplishing the goal of a desensitized state.

Intranasal lysine aspirin can also be used for aspirin challenge and similarly provokes deminished rates of lower respiratory and extrarespiratory symptoms than seen with oral protocols. In a study of 131 patients who were first challenged with lysine aspirin to confirm the diagnosis, and if negative were then challenged with oral aspirin, a small subset (12%) reacted only to the oral aspirin challenge and not to the intranasal lysine aspirin challenge. Of those who reacted to the lysine-aspirin challenge, 100% developed nasal symptoms, though only 21 (18%) developed any lower respiratory symptoms. Only 2 (<2%) developed a decrease in $FEV_1$ of more than 20%, and only 7 patients (6%) developed any symptoms outside of the respiratory tract, which included facial itching, urticaria, and mild facial angioedema, whereas no gastrointestinal symptoms were reported.[7] This finding suggests that decreasing the systemic absorption of the COX-1 inhibitor leads to decreased systemic symptoms without compromising the ability to bring about a desensitized state. Moreover, it highlights a role for both local nasal and systemic effector cells in patients with AERD.

## PATHOPHYSIOLOGY OF ASPIRIN-INDUCED REACTIONS

The breadth of clinical symptoms noted during aspirin-induced reactions parallels the breadth of the clinical spectrum seen at baseline in patients with AERD. This clinical variation among patients, even those with a disease phenotype as distinct as AERD, suggests that the precise cellular and biochemical perturbations that cause the aspirin-induced reactions may vary from patient to patient. Like many complex medical conditions, a multitude of interconnected derangements have been reported in the cellular and mediator signaling cascades in AERD (**Table 1**). The identification of a single pathologic mechanism remains elusive and frankly frustrating for those researchers who study this disease. Fortunately for researchers, clinicians, and patients with AERD, progress has been made from all angles in recent years; we currently have a sufficient framework on which to eventually build the complete story. The lipid mediators, including cysLTs and prostaglandins, and the effector cells, including mast cells (MCs) and eosinophils, of the innate immune system are the central players that, with help from platelets, trigger the dramatic physiologic changes that occur during aspirin-induced reactions.

| Table 1 | |
|---|---|
| **Mechanisms of aspirin-induced reactions** | |
| **Cells** | **Mediators** |
| • Mast cell | • CysLTs |
| ○ Acute activation during reactions | ○ Increase acutely during reactions |
| • Eosinophil/basophil | • Prostaglandin $D_2$ |
| ○ Acute influx into respiratory tissue during reactions | ○ Increases acutely in the most severe patients during reactions |
| • Platelets | • Prostaglandin $E_2$ |
| ○ Increased platelet activation and platelet-leukocyte adhesion at baseline, which may contribute to leukotriene production and reaction symptoms | ○ Often decreases during reactions |
| | • Histamine and tryptase |
| | ○ Increase acutely during reactions, especially in patients with systemic manifestations |

## Lipid Mediators

### Leukotrienes

Early assessments of biological fluids during aspirin-induced reactions revealed the aberrant production of lipid mediators, specifically the cysLTs. Using leukotriene (LT) $E_4$, the stable metabolite of the cysLTs, as a surrogate, patients with AERD demonstrate high baseline levels of cysLTs compared with healthy and aspirin-tolerant asthmatic (ATA) controls, which further increase in urine and nasal lavage during an aspirin-induced reaction. Baseline urine $LTE_4$ ($uLTE_4$) is almost 10-fold higher in AERD than in patients with ATA, and then increases 2- to 12-fold further following oral aspirin challenge in AERD.[12] CysLT levels predict symptom severity during aspirin-induced reactions,[13] and higher baseline levels of cysLTs predict the involvement of both upper and lower respiratory symptoms during a reaction.[14] The decrease in $FEV_1$ during oral aspirin challenge is associated with the degree of baseline $uLTE_4$ elevation and the extent to which $uLTE_4$ increases during reaction.[13] This excess of cysLTs at baseline and during reaction has been recapitulated in multiple studies and forms our fundamental understanding of the pathobiology of this disease. Neither the exact mechanism that triggers the overproduction of cysLTs nor their cellular sources are known, but current data supports a role for impairments in prostaglandin (PG) $E_2$ production[15] and the contributions of MC products[16,17] and of platelet-leukocyte aggregates.[18]

### Prostaglandins

In addition to the excessive production of cysLTs in AERD, it is recognized that $PGD_2$ is also overproduced. Multiple studies have demonstrated that patients with AERD have high levels of $PGD_2$ or one of the $PGD_2$ metabolites at baseline when compared with healthy and ATA controls.[19,20] These values increase on exposure to aspirin, with significant increases from baseline noted at the onset of clinical reaction in both plasma[19] and urine.[20,21] Similar to $uLTE_4$ levels, baseline urinary tetranor-PGD-M levels, one of the dominant urinary $PGD_2$ metabolites, predict the decrease in $FEV_1$ during aspirin-triggered reactions and the increase in urinary tetranor-PGD-M during reactions correlates with symptom severity.[8] Recent work established the connection between extremely high levels of $PGD_2$ during an aspirin-induced reaction and the development of extrarespiratory symptoms, specifically rash and gastrointestinal distress, including pain, nausea, and diarrhea, which can make it more difficult for patients to successfully complete their aspirin desensitization.[8] These data suggest that $PGD_2$ contributes significantly to the symptoms seen at baseline and during aspirin-induced reactions in AERD, which is not surprising when we consider the known biological effects of $PGD_2$. The $PGD_2$ metabolite 9a,11b-$PGF_2$ is bronchoconstrictive,[22] which occurs through its signaling at the T prostanoid (TP) receptor. $PGD_2$ is also a chemoattractant for eosinophils, basophils, and innate lymphoid type 2 cells through the chemokine receptor homologous molecule expressed on Th2 lymphocytes (CRTH2).[23] The increase in $PGD_2$ production during aspirin-induced reactions inversely correlates with a decrease in peripheral blood eosinophils, likely indicating chemotaxis of CRTH2$^+$ cells to the respiratory tissue.[20] Additionally, the positive correlation between nasal symptoms scores and $PGD_2$ production and the inverse correlation between $FEV_1$ and $PGD_2$ production seen during aspirin-induced reactions highlight the contribution of $PGD_2$ to reaction-induced symptoms.

Three major questions remain about $PGD_2$ generation in AERD:

1. What is the cellular source of $PGD_2$?
2. What causes the overproduction of $PGD_2$ at baseline in some patients with AERD?

3. How is $PGD_2$ being produced during aspirin-induced reactions, in the face of pharmacologic inhibition of COX-1?

The current working hypothesis is that MCs are the primary source of $PGD_2$ in AERD. This logical conclusion is built on the knowledge that $PGD_2$ is the primary COX product of MCs and that acute MC activation during aspirin-induced reactions is assumed due to the simultaneous detection of tryptase, histamine, and cysLTs, all canonical MC products.[16,17] Further support for the role of the MC in AERD is discussed later. Eosinophils, which are abundant in the local respiratory tissue, are another potential source of $PGD_2$. Eosinophils do have the relevant terminal $PGD_2$ synthase, HPGDS, but express much less *HPGDS* transcript on a per-cell basis than do MCs.[20] It has been hypothesized that the ability of cells to generate excessive amounts of $PGD_2$ during aspirin-induced reactions when the COX-1 enzyme activity is pharmacologically inhibited is related to residual COX-2 activity. However, current evidence in subjects with ATA demonstrates that COX-2 inhibition does not suppress $PGD_2$ production or its downstream metabolites,[24] suggesting that $PGD_2$ production, at least in patients with ATA, is under COX-1 enzymatic regulation. Therefore, though the mechanism of $PGD_2$ overproduction remains elusive, it is hoped that the results of human studies using selective $PGD_2$ receptor antagonists will at least provide us with more conclusive evidence for the role of $PGD_2$ in AERD.

In addition to the elevation of $PGD_2$ during aspirin-induced reactions, the suppression of COX-1-derived $PGE_2$ following aspirin ingestion may be a key component underlying aspirin-induced reactions in AERD. Impairments in all steps along the $PGE_2$ signaling pathway, including COX-2, mPGES-1, and the $EP_2$ receptor, have been reported by multiple groups on multiple tissue and cell types from subjects with AERD.[25–30] These impairments collectively are suspected to limit the ability of tissues/cells to upregulate $PGE_2$ production during times of inflammation, making patients with AERD particularly sensitive to COX-1 inhibition. Supporting these in vitro observations are 2 findings: (1) 15 minutes after bronchial aspirin challenge, $PGE_2$ levels in the bronchoalveolar lavage (BAL) decreased significantly in 11 patients with AERD[31] and (2) pretreatment with inhaled $PGE_2$ prevented the aspirin-induced increase in $uLTE_4$ and the aspirin-induced decrease in $FEV_1$ during aspirin challenge.[15] $PGE_2$ does serve as a negative regulator of 5-lipoxygenase (5-LO) through cyclic AMP/protein kinase A (PKA)[32]; an aspirin-induced decrease in $PGE_2$ production, even locally, may be one driving factor for the excessive production of 5-LO products, specifically cysLTs. However, $PGE_2$ levels measured in the urine and nasal lavage during aspirin-induced reactions remain unchanged, suggesting that $PGE_2$ is not the sole mediator responsible for these reactions. Urinary $PGE_2$ levels do not decrease during aspirin-induced reactions[8,33]; but there are significant amounts of $PGE_2$ generated in the kidney tubules, so urinary measurement may not be the best assessment of changes in respiratory $PGE_2$. In a small cohort of 5 patients with AERD, aspirin ingestion did not cause a decrease in nasal $PGE_2$ levels even when their nasal cysLT levels did go up,[34] so a simple shunting mechanism is not likely to be the complete answer.

Aspirin use, independent of disease state, has direct effects on other lipid mediators, notably thromboxane (TX) $A_2$ and prostacyclin.[35] $TXA_2$ is a potent brochoconstrictor,[36] mediating its effects through the TP receptor. Additionally, $TXA_2$ supports PKA homeostasis, which in turn is critical for $LTC_4$ synthase levels and cysLT synthesis.[37] $TXA_2$ metabolites go down during reaction in most patients with AERD,[38] but those who demonstrate excessive $PGD_2$ production during a reaction similarly demonstrate $TXA_2$ production, as measured by an increase in the urinary metabolite11-dehydro$TXB_2$.[8] The TP receptor, which mediates bronchoconstriction and through which both $PGD_2$ metabolites and $TXA_2$ signal, likely plays a key role in the lower respiratory symptoms that are so often observed during aspirin-induced respiratory reactions in patients with AERD. Early phase clinical trials of a selective TP receptor antagonist in AERD[39] are ongoing and should better inform our understanding of the importance of this signaling pathway.

## Cells

During an aspirin-induced reaction in patients with AERD, we have the ability to directly and indirectly assess changes in resident and infiltrating effector cells to inform our understanding of this inflammatory state. The role of MCs, eosinophils, basophils, and platelets have been the primary focus of current research in AERD to date; current evidence supports a role for each cell in mediator generation or migration to the respiratory tissue during aspirin-induced reactions.

### Mast cells

MCs are long-lived innate immune cells in the tissue that play a central role in AERD. In a study of 8 patients with AERD, aspirin ingestion caused an increase in nasal tryptase, histamine, and cysLTs; pretreatment with oral zileuton, an inhibitor of 5-LO, blocked both the nasal symptoms and the increase in nasal tryptase and cysLTs. This finding strongly suggests that MCs are activated during the nasal response to aspirin and that 5-LO products are important for the development of nasal symptoms and for the further release of MC mediators.[17] Tryptase and histamine can also be released systemically, but this tends to be most pronounced in patients with extrapulmonary symptoms.[40] The use of sodium cromolyn to successfully inhibit aspirin-induced reactions further emphasizes the importance of MCs.[41] However, there are no differences in the numbers of MCs within the nasal polyp tissue of patients with AERD[20]; there is no evidence that MC activation occurs through an immunoglobulin E–dependent process in AERD. Therefore, we are left to question why MC activation occurs following aspirin ingestion in AERD and not ATA or healthy controls. One possible explanation returns us to the impairment in $PGE_2$ production observed in subjects with AERD. $PGE_2$ serves as an inhibitor of MC activation,[42] and the loss of this break following the inactivation of COX-1 may lead to unfettered MC activation.

### Eosinophils/basophils

Chronic eosinophilic sinusitis is one hallmark of AERD, and eosinophils are likely drivers of the chronic inflammatory state in the respiratory tissue. Additionally, many patients with AERD demonstrate mild to moderate chronic peripheral blood eosinophilia.[20,43] Less is known about basophils in the chronic state. During an aspirin-induced reaction, an influx of both eosinophils and basophils can be demonstrated into the nose[44] and into the BAL following an inhaled aspirin challenge.[31] Correspondingly, a decrease of peripheral blood eosinophils within 1 hour of the onset of reaction symptoms following aspirin challenge has been observed.[20,38] This migration of $CRTH2^+$ cells from the blood stream to the respiratory tissue when $PGD_2$ levels are increasing suggests that the effector cells are responding to the $PGD_2$ gradient produced from within the local tissue.[20] Clearly defining the role of eosinophils and basophils as drivers of the acute reaction requires further investigation.

### Platelets

Although the major function of platelet activation is the formation of thrombi in response to vessel wall injury, platelets also influence the function and activation of immune cells and can facilitate granulocyte recruitment into sites of tissue inflammation. There is an increasing body of evidence to suggest that platelet activation may be specifically associated with the pathophysiology of AERD. Platelet activation is mediated by the binding of a diverse set of stimuli, and on activation the cell adhesion molecule P-selectin is expressed on the extracellular surface. This expression in turn facilitates platelet adhesion onto leukocytes, which constitutively express the ligand P-selectin glycoprotein ligand 1. This P-selectin–dependent adhesion to leukocytes allows for the priming and migration of these cells to inflamed tissues. Indeed studies have now shown that there is a higher percentage of platelet-adherent leukocytes in both the circulation and within the nasal polyp tissue of patients with AERD, compared with ATA controls, as well as an increased percentage of circulating platelets that express P-selectin in AERD.[18,45]

Platelets also possess a range of inflammatory mediators that are released on activation and can act as a supply of newly synthesized lipid mediators. It may be that the platelets from patients with AERD are uniquely capable of inciting inflammation. For example, when compared with platelets from ATA controls, circulating platelets from patients with AERD generate an abnormal response when stimulated with aspirin in vitro, with a release of cytotoxic mediators and free radicals.[46] Platelets from patients with AERD also produce higher quantities of lipoxygenase products than do those from patients with ATA.[47] The increased presence of platelet-adherent neutrophils in AERD[18] contributes to the overproduction of cysLTs seen in the disease, through the transcellular metabolism of arachidonic acid. Although neutrophils possess active 5-LO enzyme activity and can produce $LTA_4$ as a leukotriene intermediate, they lack the final $LTC_4$ synthase enzyme required for the production of cysLTs and cannot, on their own, convert arachidonic acid into cysLTs. Platelets lack 5-LO but do express $LTC_4$ synthase. However, when neutrophils and platelets are in close contact through P-selectin–dependent adhesion, excess $LTA_4$ released from the neutrophils can be converted into cysLTs by the platelet's $LTC_4$ synthase, creating a transcellular mechanism for the release of additional cysLTs.[18]

Additional investigations are underway to determine if the levels of platelet activation or platelet-leukocyte adhesion further increase during aspirin-induced reactions, which would provide a clear indication that platelets are directly involved in the acute reactions.

### Innate Immune Mediators

Two mediators of innate type 2 immunity, interleukin 33 (IL-33) and thymic stromal lymphopoietin (TSLP), have also recently been implicated in the pathogenesis of AERD and the aspirin-induced reactions. IL-33 and TSLP are cytokines largely derived from structural cells and are known to provide an initial response to viral infections. These cytokines can induce MC activation and eosinophil accumulation into inflamed respiratory tissues,[48,49] and nasal polyps from patients with AERD have been found to strongly express both IL-33 and TSLP.[20,50] Additionally, in a mouse model of AERD, pharmacologic blockade of either IL-33 or its receptor completely prevented the increase in lung resistance and release of MC mediators induced by inhaled aspirin challenge.[50] These early studies suggest that activation and amplification of the innate type 2 immune system may play a role in the underlying mechanisms that lead to the chronic inflammation and/or the acute aspirin-induced reactions in AERD.

### SUMMARY

There are extensive data to support that the clinical symptoms observed during acute aspirin-induced reactions in patients with AERD are largely due to both the sudden release of proinflammatory lipid mediators, particularly cysLTs and $PGD_2$, and the rapid influx of effector cells into the respiratory tissues. To date, the data also strongly suggest that these lipid mediators are primarily produced by MCs, with likely contributions by platelet-leukocyte aggregates as well. However, there are many remaining questions regarding the underlying pathophysiologic mechanisms of these reactions. Neither the primary insult that causes the initial chronic disease process to begin nor the acute trigger of aspirin-induced reactions are known. Research is underway to further elucidate the mechanisms of reaction, in the hopes that understanding more about the pathogenesis of the COX-1 inhibitor–induced reactions will guide us to a better understanding of the disease overall and to the development of better treatments for our patients.

## REFERENCES

1. Stevenson DD, Szczeklik A. Clinical and pathologic perspectives on aspirin sensitivity and asthma. J Allergy Clin Immunol 2006;118(4):773–86 [quiz: 87–8].
2. Szczeklik A, Gryglewski RJ, Czerniawska-Mysik G. Clinical patterns of hypersensitivity to nonsteroidal anti-inflammatory drugs and their pathogenesis. J Allergy Clin Immunol 1977;60(5):276–84.
3. Szczeklik A, Nizankowska E, Bochenek G, et al. Safety of a specific COX-2 inhibitor in aspirin-induced asthma. Clin Exp Allergy 2001;31(2):219–25.
4. Dahlen B, Szczeklik A, Murray JJ, Celecoxib in Aspirin-Intolerant Asthma Study Group. Celecoxib in patients with asthma and aspirin intolerance. The Celecoxib in Aspirin-Intolerant Asthma Study Group. N Engl J Med 2001;344(2):142.
5. Berges-Gimeno MP, Simon RA, Stevenson DD. Early effects of aspirin desensitization treatment in asthmatic patients with aspirin-exacerbated respiratory disease. Ann Allergy Asthma Immunol 2003;90(3):338–41.
6. Lee RU, White AA, Ding D, et al. Use of intranasal ketorolac and modified oral aspirin challenge for desensitization of aspirin-exacerbated respiratory disease. Ann Allergy Asthma Immunol 2010;105(2):130–5.
7. Miller B, Mirakian R, Gane S, et al. Nasal lysine aspirin challenge in the diagnosis of aspirin - exacerbated respiratory disease: asthma and rhinitis. Clin Exp Allergy 2013;43(8):874–80.
8. Cahill KN, Bensko JC, Boyce JA, et al. Prostaglandin D(2): a dominant mediator of aspirin-exacerbated respiratory disease. J Allergy Clin Immunol 2015;135(1): 245–52.
9. White A, Ludington E, Mehra P, et al. Effect of leukotriene modifier drugs on the safety of oral aspirin challenges. Ann Allergy Asthma Immunol 2006;97(5): 688–93.
10. Stevenson DD, Simon RA, Mathison DA, et al. Montelukast is only partially effective in inhibiting aspirin responses in aspirin-sensitive asthmatics. Ann Allergy Asthma Immunol 2000;85(6 Pt 1):477–82.
11. White A, Bigby T, Stevenson D. Intranasal ketorolac challenge for the diagnosis of aspirin-exacerbated respiratory disease. Ann Allergy Asthma Immunol 2006; 97(2):190–5.
12. Christie PE, Tagari P, Ford-Hutchinson AW, et al. Urinary leukotriene E4 concentrations increase after aspirin challenge in aspirin-sensitive asthmatic subjects. Am Rev Respir Dis 1991;143(5 Pt 1):1025–9.
13. Daffern PJ, Muilenburg D, Hugli TE, et al. Association of urinary leukotriene E4 excretion during aspirin challenges with severity of respiratory responses. J Allergy Clin Immunol 1999;104(3 Pt 1):559–64.

14. Swierczynska M, Nizankowska-Mogilnicka E, Zarychta J, et al. Nasal versus bronchial and nasal response to oral aspirin challenge: clinical and biochemical differences between patients with aspirin-induced asthma/rhinitis. J Allergy Clin Immunol 2003;112(5):995–1001.

15. Sestini P, Armetti L, Gambaro G, et al. Inhaled PGE2 prevents aspirin-induced bronchoconstriction and urinary LTE4 excretion in aspirin-sensitive asthma. Am J Respir Crit Care Med 1996;153(2):572–5.

16. Mita H, Endoh S, Kudoh M, et al. Possible involvement of mast-cell activation in aspirin provocation of aspirin-induced asthma. Allergy 2001;56(11):1061–7.

17. Fischer AR, Rosenberg MA, Lilly CM, et al. Direct evidence for a role of the mast cell in the nasal response to aspirin in aspirin-sensitive asthma. J Allergy Clin Immunol 1994;94(6 Pt 1):1046–56.

18. Laidlaw TM, Kidder MS, Bhattacharyya N, et al. Cysteinyl leukotriene overproduction in aspirin-exacerbated respiratory disease is driven by platelet-adherent leukocytes. Blood 2012;119(16):3790–8.

19. Bochenek G, Nagraba K, Nizankowska E, et al. A controlled study of 9alpha,11beta-PGF2 (a prostaglandin D2 metabolite) in plasma and urine of patients with bronchial asthma and healthy controls after aspirin challenge. J Allergy Clin Immunol 2003;111(4):743–9.

20. Buchheit KM, Cahill KN, Katz HR, et al. Thymic stromal lymphopoietin controls prostaglandin D2 generation in patients with aspirin-exacerbated respiratory disease. J Allergy Clin Immunol 2016;137(5):1566–76.e5.

21. Higashi N, Mita H, Ono E, et al. Profile of eicosanoid generation in aspirin-intolerant asthma and anaphylaxis assessed by new biomarkers. J Allergy Clin Immunol 2010;125(5):1084–91.e6.

22. Beasley CR, Robinson C, Featherstone RL, et al. 9 alpha,11 beta-prostaglandin F2, a novel metabolite of prostaglandin D2 is a potent contractile agonist of human and guinea pig airways. J Clin Invest 1987;79(3):978–83.

23. Monneret G, Gravel S, Diamond M, et al. Prostaglandin D2 is a potent chemoattractant for human eosinophils that acts via a novel DP receptor. Blood 2001; 98(6):1942–8.

24. Daham K, James A, Balgoma D, et al. Effects of selective COX-2 inhibition on allergen-induced bronchoconstriction and airway inflammation in asthma. J Allergy Clin Immunol 2014;134(2):306–13.

25. Roca-Ferrer J, Garcia-Garcia FJ, Pereda J, et al. Reduced expression of COXs and production of prostaglandin E(2) in patients with nasal polyps with or without aspirin-intolerant asthma. J Allergy Clin Immunol 2011;128(1):66–72.e1.

26. Ying S, Meng Q, Scadding G, et al. Aspirin-sensitive rhinosinusitis is associated with reduced E-prostanoid 2 receptor expression on nasal mucosal inflammatory cells. J Allergy Clin Immunol 2006;117(2):312–8.

27. Corrigan CJ, Napoli RL, Meng Q, et al. Reduced expression of the prostaglandin E2 receptor E-prostanoid 2 on bronchial mucosal leukocytes in patients with aspirin-sensitive asthma. J Allergy Clin Immunol 2012;129(6):1636–46.

28. Adamusiak AM, Stasikowska-Kanicka O, Lewandowska-Polak A, et al. Expression of arachidonate metabolism enzymes and receptors in nasal polyps of aspirin-hypersensitive asthmatics. Int Arch Allergy Immunol 2012;157(4):354–62.

29. Laidlaw TM, Cutler AJ, Kidder MS, et al. Prostaglandin E2 resistance in granulocytes from patients with aspirin-exacerbated respiratory disease. J Allergy Clin Immunol 2014;133(6):1692–701.e3.

30. Cahill KN, Raby BA, Zhou X, et al. Impaired EP expression causes resistance to prostaglandin E in nasal polyp fibroblasts from subjects with AERD. Am J Respir Cell Mol Biol 2016;54(1):34–40.
31. Szczeklik A, Sladek K, Dworski R, et al. Bronchial aspirin challenge causes specific eicosanoid response in aspirin-sensitive asthmatics. Am J Respir Crit Care Med 1996;154(6 Pt 1):1608–14.
32. Flamand N, Surette ME, Picard S, et al. Cyclic AMP-mediated inhibition of 5-lipoxygenase translocation and leukotriene biosynthesis in human neutrophils. Mol Pharmacol 2002;62(2):250–6.
33. Mastalerz L, Sanak M, Gawlewicz-Mroczka A, et al. Prostaglandin E2 systemic production in patients with asthma with and without aspirin hypersensitivity. Thorax 2008;63(1):27–34.
34. Ferreri NR, Howland WC, Stevenson DD, et al. Release of leukotrienes, prostaglandins, and histamine into nasal secretions of aspirin-sensitive asthmatics during reaction to aspirin. Am Rev Respir Dis 1988;137(4):847–54.
35. Kyrle PA, Eichler HG, Jager U, et al. Inhibition of prostacyclin and thromboxane A2 generation by low-dose aspirin at the site of plug formation in man in vivo. Circulation 1987;75(5):1025–9.
36. Takami M, Tsukada W. Correlative alteration of thromboxane A2 with antigen-induced bronchoconstriction and the role of platelets as a source of TXA2 synthesis in guinea pigs: effect of DP-1904, an inhibitor of thromboxane synthetase. Pharmacol Res 1998;38(2):133–9.
37. Tornhamre S, Ehnhage A, Kolbeck KG, et al. Uncoupled regulation of leukotriene C4 synthase in platelets from aspirin-intolerant asthmatics and healthy volunteers after aspirin treatment. Clin Exp Allergy 2002;32(11):1566–73.
38. Sladek K, Szczeklik A. Cysteinyl leukotrienes overproduction and mast cell activation in aspirin-provoked bronchospasm in asthma. Eur Respir J 1993;6(3):391–9.
39. Health NIo. Trial to determine the safety of oral ifetroban in patients with a history of aspirin exacerbated respiratory disease. 2015. Available at: https://clinicaltrials.gov/ct2/show/NCT02216357?term=AERD&rank=7. Accessed December 23, 2015.
40. Bosso JV, Schwartz LB, Stevenson DD. Tryptase and histamine release during aspirin-induced respiratory reactions. J Allergy Clin Immunol 1991;88(6):830–7.
41. Basomba A, Romar A, Pelaez A, et al. The effect of sodium cromoglycate in preventing aspirin induced bronchospasm. Clin Allergy 1976;6(3):269–75.
42. Kay LJ, Yeo WW, Peachell PT. Prostaglandin E2 activates EP2 receptors to inhibit human lung mast cell degranulation. Br J Pharmacol 2006;147(7):707–13.
43. Bochenek G, Kuschill-Dziurda J, Szafraniec K, et al. Certain subphenotypes of aspirin-exacerbated respiratory disease distinguished by latent class analysis. J Allergy Clin Immunol 2014;133(1):98–103.e1–6.
44. Kupczyk M, Kurmanowska Z, Kuprys-Lipinska I, et al. Mediators of inflammation in nasal lavage from aspirin intolerant patients after aspirin challenge. Respir Med 2010;104(10):1404–9.
45. Mitsui C, Kajiwara K, Hayashi H, et al. Platelet activation markers overexpressed specifically in patients with aspirin-exacerbated respiratory disease. J Allergy Clin Immunol 2016;137(2):400–11.
46. Ameisen JC, Capron A, Joseph M, et al. Aspirin-sensitive asthma: abnormal platelet response to drugs inducing asthmatic attacks. Diagnostic and physiopathological implications. Int Arch Allergy Appl Immunol 1985;78(4):438–48.
47. Plaza V, Prat J, Rosello J, et al. In vitro release of arachidonic acid metabolites, glutathione peroxidase, and oxygen-free radicals from platelets of asthmatic patients with and without aspirin intolerance. Thorax 1995;50(5):490–6.

48. Kumar RK, Foster PS, Rosenberg HF. Respiratory viral infection, epithelial cytokines, and innate lymphoid cells in asthma exacerbations. J Leukoc Biol 2014; 96(3):391–6.
49. Iwasaki A, Medzhitov R. Control of adaptive immunity by the innate immune system. Nat Immunol 2015;16(4):343–53.
50. Liu T, Kanaoka Y, Barrett NA, et al. Aspirin-exacerbated respiratory disease involves a cysteinyl leukotriene-driven IL-33-mediated mast cell activation pathway. J Immunol 2015;195(8):3537–45.

# Performing Aspirin Desensitization in Aspirin-Exacerbated Respiratory Disease

Jeremy D. Waldram, MD, Ronald A. Simon, MD*

## KEYWORDS

- Aspirin • Desensitization • AERD • AERD treatment • AERD diagnosis

## KEY POINTS

- Aspirin desensitization followed by daily aspirin therapy is an important treatment modality in aspirin-exacerbated respiratory disease (AERD) and should be used by allergists.
- Aspirin challenge/desensitization in patients with AERD is a provocative test that will likely induce symptoms, although pretreatment can attenuate the symptom severity.
- Despite being a provocative test, aspirin challenge/desensitization can be performed safely in an outpatient setting in most patients with AERD.

## INTRODUCTION

Aspirin-exacerbated respiratory disease (AERD) is characterized by chronic rhinosinusitis with nasal polyposis (CRSwNP), asthma, and intolerance to cyclooxygenase-1 (COX-1) inhibiting medications. In patients with AERD, aspirin and other COX-1 blocking medications produce reactions involving the upper and/or lower airways within minutes to hours of ingestion.

The reactions to these medications in AERD are categorized as pseudoallergy because they result from an abnormal biochemical response to the pharmacologic actions of these medications rather than from an immunologically mediated process. The reactions, however, can be severe.

Nonsteroidal antiinflammatory drug (NSAID) challenge is the method of confirming a suspected AERD diagnosis. NSAID desensitization followed by daily aspirin therapy is a well-documented treatment option for AERD. This article focuses specifically on performing NSAID challenge and desensitization in this patient population.

Disclosure statement: The authors have nothing to disclose.
Department of Allergy and Immunology, Scripps Clinic Carmel Valley, Scripps Clinic, 3811 Valley Centre Drive, Suite 4A, San Diego, CA 92130, USA
* Corresponding author.
E-mail address: Simon.ronald@scrippshealth.org

Immunol Allergy Clin N Am 36 (2016) 693–703
http://dx.doi.org/10.1016/j.iac.2016.06.006
immunology.theclinics.com
0889-8561/16/$ – see front matter © 2016 Elsevier Inc. All rights reserved.

## CHALLENGE VERSUS DESENSITIZATION

Graded drug challenge, or test dosing, entails cautious administration of increasing doses of a medication. Such challenges involve few steps and are not intended to induce drug tolerance. They are typically performed to exclude the diagnosis of immediate drug hypersensitivity in patients considered to have low pretest probability based on history.

Drug desensitization, also referred to as temporary induction of drug tolerance, is performed when there is a high likelihood of drug hypersensitivity and the medication is necessary for patients. Desensitization is designed to temporarily alter the patients' response to a drug to allow patients to take it without adverse reaction. Drug desensitization protocols call for the administration of incremental doses of a drug over time until the drug can be safely taken without adverse reaction.[1]

Both graded challenge and desensitization are used in the diagnosis and treatment of AERD. Graded challenge may be performed alone in order to simply confirm or refute the diagnosis of AERD. However, challenge and desensitization are routinely combined in AERD for diagnostic and therapeutic purposes; these terms are often used interchangeably.

## OVERVIEW OF NONSTEROIDAL ANTIINFLAMMATORY DRUG CHALLENGE IN ASPIRIN-EXACERBATED RESPIRATORY DISEASE
### Purpose

NSAID challenges in the context of AERD are used to diagnose NSAID pseudoallergy. In contrast to most drug challenges, NSAID challenge in a patient suspected of having AERD is a provocative challenge, meaning it is likely to produce a reaction. It is done with the goal of confirming the diagnosis of AERD, whereas drug challenge in other situations is typically done only on patients not thought to have drug allergy or sensitivity.

### Safety

Given the fact that NSAID challenges in AERD are likely to cause symptoms, the following measures warrant attention:

- Informed consent is essential.
- Patients should be optimized in terms of asthma control as discussed later.
- Patients should receive pretreatment as discussed later.
- The challenge should be done in the appropriate setting. In most cases, an outpatient allergy clinic will suffice; but there may be patients that require more intensive monitoring. Clinical judgment is warranted to determine the appropriate location for challenge.
- Historically, intravenous access was obtained as part of the challenge procedure; but this is not standard practice at the authors' institution. There may be situations in which an individual clinician might want to have intravenous access.

### Prechallenge Considerations

Pretreating patients with suspected AERD before NSAID challenge is helpful in mitigating the risk of a severe reaction.

A leukotriene-modifying drug (LTMD) should be started before the challenge if patients are not already taking one, as evidence supports their ability to dampen the reaction during challenge.[2–5] Patients on LTMD premedication tend to have less severe bronchospasm during challenge as compared with patients not on LTMD premedication. One study showed a 90% reduction in asthmatic reactions to aspirin challenge with montelukast premedication.[6] In addition, nasal and ocular symptoms remain despite LTMD use, which is important because the goal is to identify NSAID sensitivity.[6] Challenges carried out before LTMD use often resulted in severe asthmatic symptoms, which prevented physicians from performing them in the outpatient setting.

Leukotriene receptor blockers montelukast and zafirlukast have been shown to not completely mask the upper respiratory symptoms during oral NSAID challenge[3,6]; they are, thus, the preferred LTMDs to use. Zileuton, a 5-lipoxygenase inhibitor, has not been studied as rigorously in this context; but one small study showed that it did not mask symptoms completely in 6 out of 6 patients.[7] The potential disadvantage of using zileuton as pretreatment is a false-negative result.

The authors' practice is to prescribe montelukast 10 mg daily starting 3 days before the challenge or 10 mg twice a day for 1 day before the challenge and then 10 mg daily on each day of the challenge. Alternatively, one may use extended release zileuton 1200 mg twice daily for at least 3 days before the challenge.

Patients are encouraged to continue topical corticosteroids before and during the challenge, which includes inhaled (with or without long-acting beta agonists) and intranasal corticosteroids. The authors prefer that asthmatic patients are taking a combination inhaled steroid/long-acting beta agonist at the time of challenge.

There is no indication to use cromolyn or antihistamines as premedication. H1 blockers blunted reactions to aspirin in one study,[8] and cromolyn delayed the onset of symptoms in another.[9] Blunting the reaction completely defeats the purpose of the challenge. Delaying the onset of symptoms may lead to a more severe reaction as an additional dose of medication may be given while a reaction is already pending. Therefore, these medications are not recommended as part of the premedication plan. In fact, patients are requested to stop them a week before challenge if already taking them.

It is also important to ensure patients' asthma is optimally treated before the challenge. A prebronchodilator forced expiratory volume in the first second of expiration ($FEV_1$) greater than or equal to 60% of predicted and within 10% of the patients' best is recommended.[10] Some patients will need a course of systemic corticosteroids in order to prepare them adequately for the challenge. Systemic corticosteroids do not mask reactions to NSAIDs in patients with AERD or do so to a minimal extent; it is, therefore, acceptable for patients to be taking them at the time of the challenge.[3]

## TYPES OF NONSTEROIDAL ANTIINFLAMMATORY DRUG CHALLENGES IN ASPIRIN-EXACERBATED RESPIRATORY DISEASE

Oral and inhalational agents have been used for NSAID challenge, and both are effective.

Aspirin is the most common oral medication used. It is widely available, cheap, and has not been implicated in any confirmed cases of immunoglobulin E–mediated reactions, including anaphylaxis. Furthermore, there is more experience with aspirin than with any other NSAID, as it has been the most common drug used in NSAID challenges in the published literature.

Parenteral ketorolac (Toradol) can be diluted in saline and administered intranasally as an NSAID challenge to diagnose AERD.[10] A study of 100 patients evaluated nasal ketorolac in conjunction with oral aspirin in a challenge/desensitization protocol.[11] During the first 4 steps of the protocol, patients received increasing doses of intranasal ketorolac at 30-minute intervals. Most patients reacted during the intranasal portion of the procedure, suggesting that ketorolac is effective as a means of NSAID challenge in these patients. In countries outside the United States, aspirin-lysine is available for bronchial or nasal inhalation.[12] Similar to ketorolac challenge, the procedure involves administering increasing doses of aspirin-lysine at 30-minute intervals.

Ketorolac and aspirin-lysine have advantages and disadvantages in NSAID challenge in AERD. The advantages of using these agents are listed here:

- Symptoms induced by bronchial or nasal challenge tend to be less severe and more quickly reversible relative to oral challenges.
- Bronchial/nasal challenges are more convenient for both patients and provider, as they can be performed more quickly.
- Nasal administration is safer for patients whose $FEV_1$ precludes oral challenge.

The disadvantages to bronchial/nasal challenge include the following:

- There is some evidence that challenge with these agents may be less sensitive as compared with oral challenge, thus, leading to potential false-negative results.[13,14]
- Aspirin-lysine is not available in the United States.
- Nasal inhalation cannot be done in patients with complete or severe nasal obstruction secondary to polyposis.

## NONSTEROIDAL ANTIINFLAMMATORY DRUG CHALLENGE PROTOCOLS IN ASPIRIN-EXACERBATED RESPIRATORY DISEASE
### Procedures

Aspirin is the preferred medication for NSAID challenge in AERD. Commercially available aspirin tablets may be used, and lower doses can be obtained by using a pill cutter. The typical starting dose of aspirin is 40.5 mg, but this may be halved in patients at higher risk of severe reactions. This starting dose is based on a study that showed most patients with AERD will react after a dose of 45 or 60 mg.[15] The aspirin dose is doubled every 3 hours until a dose of 325 mg is given or patients have a reaction. The challenge is completed in 1 or 2 days.

There is some debate regarding the optimal interval between doses. Some experts suggest that 90 minutes is sufficient unless patients specifically report symptoms starting 90 minutes after ingestion during previous reactions.[10] It is the authors' practice to wait 3 hours between the higher doses and 90 minutes between the lower doses of aspirin. Dosing intervals less than 90 minutes may lead to the administration of another dose while a reaction is pending.

The authors do not typically use placebos in NSAID challenge when performed for the purpose of confirming an AERD diagnosis in patients with high pretest probability based on history. However, placebo doses are useful in certain situations, such as research studies and when patients are not suspected of having NSAID sensitivity.

Ketorolac may also be used for challenge in AERD by following the first 4 steps in the ketorolac/aspirin desensitization protocol used at the authors' institution (Table 1).

Various aspirin-lysine protocols have been used outside the United States.[16,17] The reader may refer to the references cited for more detailed information on these protocols if desired.

| Table 1 | |
|---|---|
| **Nasal ketorolac and oral aspirin challenge protocol** | |
| **Time** | **Dose of Ketorolac[a] (in mg) or Oral Aspirin (in mg)** |
| Day 1 | |
| 8:00 AM | Ketorolac 1.26 (1 spray in one nostril) |
| 8:30 AM | Ketorolac 2.52 (1 spray in each nostril) |
| 9:00 AM | Ketorolac 5.04 (2 sprays in each nostril) |
| 9:30 AM | Ketorolac 7.56 (3 sprays in each nostril) |
| 10:30 AM | Aspirin 60 |
| 12:00 PM | Aspirin 60 |
| 3:00 PM | Instructions and discharge |
| Day 2 | |
| 8:00 AM | Aspirin 150 |
| 11:00 AM | Aspirin 325 |
| 2:00 PM | Instructions and discharge |

Clinical and objective evaluation performed every 30 minutes and as needed.
[a] Prepared by mixing ketorolac 60 mg/2 mL with normal saline 2.75 mL and then placing it in a nasal spray bottle that delivers 100 µL/actuation; each spray will now actuate 1.26 mg of ketorolac.

## Interpreting the Results

Typical reactions to oral or nasal NSAID challenge include the following[11]:

- Conjunctivitis or rhinitis (naso-ocular reaction)
- A decrease in nasal flow rate by 20% or more
- Lower airway symptoms or signs (bronchospasm; decrease in $FEV_1$ by 15% or more)
- Laryngospasm
- Systemic response (gastrointestinal pain, flushing, urticaria, and rarely, hypotension)

Patients not uncommonly have a combination of the reactions described earlier. A classic reaction involves naso-ocular and lower respiratory symptoms, including a decline in $FEV_1$ by 15% or more.

A positive aspirin-lysine bronchial challenge is defined as a decrease in $FEV_1$ by 20% or more.[13,14] Bronchospasm is typically the only reaction in bronchial challenge. It usually occurs around 20 minutes and is rapidly reversed with inhaled beta agonists.[13,14]

Patients with a positive challenge are diagnosed with AERD and treated accordingly. Patients with a negative challenge either do not have AERD or the symptoms were masked by premedication, namely, LTMDs. The procedure should be repeated off of LTMDs to evaluate for the latter scenario, especially when the clinical history is highly supportive of AERD. If desensitization was scheduled to be done at the same time as the challenge, the physician may wish to proceed with it as a matter of convenience to the patients. This topic is discussed in more detail later.

## Management of Symptoms During Challenge

As mentioned previously, LTMDs dramatically reduce reaction severity; but symptoms will usually still occur if patients have AERD, and they may last several hours. Recommendations for treatment are as follows[10]:

- Ocular symptoms may be treated with an oral or ocular antihistamine.
- Nasal symptoms, such as congestion, may be treated with topical nasal decongestants or corticosteroids. Oral or nasal antihistamines may be helpful as well.
- Bronchospasm may be treated with a short-acting bronchodilator, such as albuterol, as needed to relieve symptoms.
- Laryngospasm may be treated with nebulized racemic epinephrine and/or intramuscular epinephrine depending on the severity.
- Gastrointestinal symptoms (nausea, vomiting, abdominal pain) are not common but do occur and can be severe. These symptoms may be treated with oral or intravenous H2 blockers or antiemetics.
- Systemic reactions, although very rare, should be treated with intramuscular epinephrine and intravenous fluids as needed.

## OVERVIEW OF NONSTEROIDAL ANTIINFLAMMATORY DRUG DESENSITIZATION IN ASPIRIN-EXACERBATED RESPIRATORY DISEASE
### Purpose

As mentioned previously, desensitization is used to induce a temporary state of tolerance to a medication. The medication must be taken routinely following desensitization or tolerance will be lost.

Aspirin desensitization followed by daily aspirin administration is used therapeutically in AERD in many patients. Numerous studies have demonstrated the beneficial effect of this treatment modality. Although a full description of the evidence supporting aspirin desensitization in AERD is outside the scope of this article, a list of some of the benefits documented in the literature[18–21] is provided:

- Overall improvement in quality of life
- Improvement in sense of smell
- Improvement in nasal and asthma symptom scores
- Decreased rate of polyp growth and, thus, need for sinus surgery
- Decreased need for systemic corticosteroids
- Less frequent/severe sinus infections

In patients with AERD, one should consider aspirin desensitization for the following reasons[10,22]:

- CRSwNP that is refractory to topical corticosteroids and other therapies; less robust evidence for improvement in asthma symptoms
- Need for aspirin in the setting of cardiovascular disease
- Need for NSAIDs to treat chronic inflammatory conditions, such as rheumatic disease

### Safety

Aspirin desensitization carries the same risks as aspirin challenge described earlier and, therefore, warrants the same precautions.

Historically, aspirin desensitization was performed in hospital settings, often in the intensive care unit. Premedication, as discussed earlier, has decreased the need for intensive monitoring in most cases. In addition, the use of inhalational medication in combination with aspirin has decreased the severity of reactions in most cases and has essentially shifted them from the lower to the upper airway. Some patients, based on asthma severity, other comorbidities, or per clinician preference, may undergo inpatient desensitization; but most desensitization procedures may be safely carried out in an appropriately equipped allergy clinic. The authors' institution has performed hundreds of NSAID challenge/desensitization procedures in the outpatient setting without any hospitalizations or deaths.

### Predesensitization Considerations

Aspirin desensitization shares many of the same considerations as the NSAID challenge described earlier. Some additional items are worthy of mention:

- Appropriate patient selection is important. Desensitization, although relatively safe, is not without risk. It typically requires a 2-day commitment from patients and should only be done for patients likely to benefit from it.
- A history of a previous severe reaction to an NSAID does not exclude patients from desensitization. The severity of historical reactions does not predict reaction severity during desensitization.[15]
- Optimal treatment of pertinent comorbidities is helpful. These comorbidities include allergic rhinitis, acid reflux, and sinus/bronchial infections.
- Sinus debulking surgery should be performed before desensitization if needed. Aspirin therapy has not been shown to have a significant impact on polyp tissue already present at the time of desensitization.[23] Therefore, surgery should be done 2 to 4 weeks before desensitization to maximize the benefit and to avoid the need for aspirin cessation during the perioperative period, which will require a repeat desensitization. Polyps in patients who have had a prior debulking surgery may respond well to a course of systemic corticosteroids, and this medical debulking may also be used before desensitization.

## NONSTEROIDAL ANTIINFLAMMATORY DRUG DESENSITIZATION PROTOCOLS IN ASPIRIN-EXACERBATED RESPIRATORY DISEASE
### Procedures

Historically, a 3-day oral aspirin desensitization protocol was standard, with intervals of 3 hours between doses.[24] Although cumbersome, with an average time to discharge of 2.6 days,[25] the protocol allowed for sufficient time between doses to identify a reaction, thus, eliminating the possibility of adding an additional dose just as a reaction is about to occur. Premedication with LTMDs significantly changed the desensitization process, and most patients will not require 3 days for desensitization.

The NSAID desensitization protocol used at the authors' institution involves ketorolac and oral aspirin (see **Table 1**). Each ketorolac dose is separated by a 30-minute interval, whereas each aspirin dose is separated by a 3-hour interval. The exceptions to these time periods are the final ketorolac dose and the initial aspirin doses. A 60-minute interval separates the final ketorolac dose from the first aspirin dose, and a 90-minute interval is used between the first and second doses of 60 mg of aspirin.

Spirometry, nasal inspiratory flow, and symptom scores are monitored at regular intervals during the desensitization protocol. When a reaction occurs, patients' symptoms are treated and the procedure resumes. The dose that elicited the reaction is repeated until the patients no longer react to it. At that point, one can proceed to the next step in the protocol and continue in like manner until patients have ingested a full 325-mg dose without developing symptoms.

Using this protocol, most patients will react to ketorolac and are typically desensitized after the first day. Doses of 150 and 325 mg of aspirin are given on the second day to ensure completion of desensitization. The average time to discharge is 1.9 days.[25] Another commonly used protocol is similar to the one just described but without the use of ketorolac.[10]

More recently, Chen and colleagues[26] published an article describing a new oral aspirin challenge protocol. The significant difference in this protocol is the time interval between doses. A 1-hour dose-escalation protocol was used, and nasal ketorolac was not used.

The reader may refer to the article for a complete review of the protocol, but some of the key findings are summarized here:

- Eligible patients reported a history of reacting to aspirin within an hour of exposure or had never been exposed to it.
- Fifty-seven patients underwent the 1-hour dose-escalation protocol.
- Forty-nine of the patients (86%) reacted during the desensitization, 48 of whom were able to complete the protocol. A single patient required epinephrine and was unable to finish.
- More than 96% of the patients were pretreated with an LTMD.
- The average time to reaction was 50.3 minutes after receiving the provoking dose, and the average provoking dose of aspirin was 157.4 mg.
- Twenty-three of the patients (40.3%) completed the protocol in a single day (that number includes nonreactors). The remainder of those completing the protocol did so in 2 days.
- The average time to discharge was 1.6 days.

The new oral aspirin challenge protocol proposed by Chen and colleagues[26] certainly addresses one of the main barriers to aspirin desensitization, which is time. A shorter duration of desensitization is certainly desirable to patients and providers alike.

However, there are some concerns about a 1-hour dose-escalation protocol. First, only patients reporting historical reactions occurring within an hour of exposure were included. Relying on patient recall may not be completely accurate, and recall bias is certainly a possibility. There is no evidence to support using the protocol in patients not able to provide such history, which may include many patients.

Additional issues include the relatively small number of patients that underwent the 1-hour dose-escalation protocol, the average time to onset of reactions, and the average provoking dose in the study.

The average time to onset of reaction was less than that previously published,[26] and the average provoking dose was higher compared with prior studies.[26] It is possible that the 57 patients in this study are not representative of the AERD population as a whole. There is concern that a potentially severe reactor will receive additional doses of aspirin while a reaction is already pending, thus, possibly producing severe bronchospasm. Clinical judgment and careful consideration on a case-by-case basis are certainly prudent. The 1-hour dose-escalation protocol may be a viable option for selected patients, but more data are necessary before recommending it without some reservation.

A comparison of the aforementioned protocols is found in **Table 2**.[27]

### Interpreting the Results

Interpreting the results of the NSAID challenge is discussed previously, and the same criteria are used to interpret the results of NSAID desensitization.

However, as mentioned previously, the physician may encounter a negative challenge in patients with a high pretest probability of AERD. Repeating the challenge off of premedication with LTMDs in this scenario is recommended.[28] If the procedure was done to both diagnose and desensitize patients (a combination challenge/desensitization), a practical approach is to proceed with the desensitization and start

**Table 2**
A comparison of the University of Texas Southwestern protocol with the Scripps ketorolac and 3-day oral aspirin challenge protocols

| Reactions and Timing | SW (N = 48) | Ketorolac (N = 82) | 3-d OAC (N = 92) |
|---|---|---|---|
| Naso-ocular | 30 (62%) | 54 (65%) | 35 (38%) |
| Bronchial | 36 (75%) | 26 (32%) | 35 (38%) |
| Laryngeal | 0 (0%) | 6 (7%) | 17 (19%) |
| Cutaneous | 4 (6%) | 5 (6%) | 9 (10%) |
| Gastrointestinal | 6 (13%) | 10 (12%) | 30 (33%) |
| Number of patients desensitized in 1 d | 14 (29%) | 0 (0%) | 0 (0%) |
| Number of patients desensitized in 2 d | 47 (98%) | 68 (83%) | 18 (38%) |
| Achieving desensitization in days (mean) | 1.6 | 1.9 | 2.6 |

*Abbreviations:* OAC, oral aspirin challenge; SW, University of Texas Southwestern.
*Modified from* Stevenson D, White A. Aspirin desensitization in aspirin-exacerbated respiratory disease: a consideration of a new oral challenge protocol. J Allergy Clin Immunol Pract 2015;3:932; with permission.

patients on daily aspirin. A 3-month trial should help elucidate whether aspirin is beneficial in these patients and whether to continue it.

## Management of Symptoms During Desensitization

Management of symptoms during desensitization is identical to the NSAID challenge. However, it is important to keep in mind that the goal of the challenge is to determine whether sensitivity to NSAIDs exists, whereas the goal of desensitization is to enable patients to tolerate the medication. Desensitization, therefore, requires treating through symptoms in order to get patients to the next step in the protocol. This management requires clinical judgment in deciding when patients are ready to proceed. As mentioned previously, the authors recommend repeating the dose that caused symptoms as a safety measure.

## Additional Considerations

A few additional considerations are worth noting:

- Virtually all patients with AERD can be desensitized to NSAIDs.
- Tolerating 325 mg of aspirin indicates patients will tolerate other NSAIDs and can use them as needed. Tolerance will remain as long as 325 mg of aspirin or the equivalent of another COX-1 inhibiting NSAID is taken without an interruption of more than 48 to 72 hours.
- Patients with AERD who take only 81 mg of aspirin daily will be able to remain tolerant of that dose but may not tolerate higher doses or be cross-desensitized to other NSAIDs.
- Evidence suggests that among aspirin responders, both 325 mg twice daily and 650 mg twice daily are effective in treating AERD. One study showed that about half of patients started on 650 mg twice daily were able to decrease to 325 mg twice daily with adequate control.[29] Lower doses may provide benefit in some patients, but doses as low as 100 mg daily seem to be insufficient and did not decrease side effects.[30] It is the authors' practice to start patients on 650 mg

twice daily and to follow up after 3 to 6 months. Those responding well could have their dose lowered in an attempt to find the lowest effective dose.

• Gastric irritation is the most common reason for aspirin discontinuation. The possibility of this side effect should be discussed with patients before desensitization.

## SUMMARY

NSAID challenge and desensitization are important tools in the diagnosis and treatment of AERD. Premedication and detailed protocols have made these procedures relatively safe, and they are routinely performed in allergy clinics. More data on AERD and NSAID challenge/desensitization will allow for further tailoring of the protocols in order to maximize efficiency and benefit while minimizing risk.

## REFERENCES

1. Solensky R, Khan D, Bernstein IL, et al. Drug allergy: an updated practice parameter. Ann Allergy Asthma Immunol 2010;105:273.
2. Lee DK, Haggart K, Robb F, et al. Montelukast protects against nasal lysine-aspirin challenge in patients with aspirin-induced asthma. Eur Respir J 2004; 24:226.
3. White A, Stevenson D, Simon R. The blocking effect of essential controller medications during aspirin challenges in patients with aspirin-exacerbated respiratory disease. Ann Allergy Asthma Immunol 2005;95:330.
4. Berges-Gimeno M, Simon R, Stevenson D. The effect of leukotriene-modifier drugs on aspirin-induced asthma and rhinitis reactions. Clin Exp Allergy 2002; 32:1491.
5. White A, Ludington E, Mehra P, et al. Effect of leukotriene modifier drugs on the safety of oral aspirin challenges. Ann Allergy Asthma Immunol 2006;97:688.
6. Stevenson D, Simon R, Mathison D, et al. Montelukast is only partially effective in inhibiting aspirin responses in aspirin-sensitive asthmatics. Ann Allergy Asthma Immunol 2000;85:477.
7. Pauls J, Simon R, Daffern P, et al. Lack of effect of the 5-lipoxygenase inhibitor zileuton in blocking oral aspirin challenges in aspirin-sensitive asthmatics. Ann Allergy Asthma Immunol 2000;85:40.
8. Szczeklik A, Serwonska M. Inhibition of idiosyncratic reactions to aspirin in asthmatic patients by clemastine. Thorax 1979;34:654.
9. Dahl R. Oral and inhaled sodium cromoglycate in challenge test with food allergens or acetylsalicylic acid. Allergy 1981;36:161.
10. Macy E, Bernstein J, Castells M, et al. Aspirin challenge and desensitization for aspirin-exacerbated respiratory disease: a practice paper. Ann Allergy Asthma Immunol 2007;98:172.
11. Lee RU, White AA, Ding D, et al. Use of intranasal ketorolac and modified oral aspirin challenge for desensitization of aspirin-exacerbated respiratory disease. Ann Allergy Asthma Immunol 2010;105:130.
12. Casadevall J, Ventura PJ, Mullol J, et al. Intranasal challenge with aspirin in the diagnosis of aspirin intolerant asthma: evaluation of nasal response by acoustic rhinometry. Thorax 2000;55:921.
13. Dahlen B, Zetterstrom O. Comparison of bronchial and per oral provocation with aspirin in aspirin-sensitive asthmatics. Eur Respir J 1990;3:527.

14. Nizankowska E, Bestynska-Krypel A, Cmiel A, et al. Oral and bronchial provocation tests with aspirin for diagnosis of aspirin-induced asthma. Eur Respir J 2000; 15:863.
15. Hope A, Woessner K, Simon R, et al. Rational approach to aspirin dosing during oral challenges and desensitization of patients with aspirin-exacerbated respiratory disease. J Allergy Clin Immunol 2009;123:406.
16. Milewski M, Mastalerz L, Nizankowska E, et al. Nasal provocation test with lysine-aspirin for diagnosis of aspirin-sensitive asthma. J Allergy Clin Immunol 1998; 101:581.
17. Alonso-Llamazares A, Martinez-Cocera C, Dominguez-Ortega J, et al. Nasal provocation test (NPT) with aspirin: a sensitive and safe method to diagnose aspirin-induced asthma (AIA). Allergy 2002;57:632.
18. Berges-Gimeno M, Simon R, Stevenson D. Long-term treatment with aspirin desensitization in asthmatic patients with aspirin-exacerbated respiratory disease. J Allergy Clin Immunol 2003;111:180.
19. Stevenson D, Hankammer M, Mathison D, et al. Aspirin desensitization treatment of aspirin-sensitive patients with rhinosinusitis-asthma: long-term outcomes. J Allergy Clin Immunol 1996;98:751.
20. Havel M, Ertl L, Braunschweig F, et al. Sinonasal outcome under aspirin desensitization following functional endoscopic sinus surgery in patients with aspirin triad. Eur Arch Otorhinolaryngol 2012;270:571.
21. Cho K, Soudry E, Psaltis A, et al. Long-term sinonasal outcomes of aspirin desensitization in aspirin exacerbated respiratory disease. Otolaryngol Head Neck Surg 2014;151:575.
22. Stevenson D, Simon R. Selection of patients for aspirin desensitization treatment. J Allergy Clin Immunol 2006;118:801.
23. Woessner K, White A. Evidence-based approach to aspirin desensitization in aspirin-exacerbated respiratory disease. J Allergy Clin Immunol 2013;133:286.
24. Stevenson D. Oral challenge, aspirin, NSAID, tartrazine, and sulfites. N Engl Reg Allergy Proc 1984;5:111.
25. White A, Bibgy T, Stevenson D. Use of ketorolac nasal spray in the diagnosis of aspirin-exacerbated respiratory disease. Ann Allergy Asthma Immunol 2006;97:88.
26. Chen J, Buchmiller B, Khan D. An hourly dose-escalation desensitization protocol for aspirin-exacerbated respiratory disease. J Allergy Clin Immunol Pract 2015;3:926.
27. Stevenson D, White A. Aspirin desensitization in aspirin-exacerbated respiratory disease: a consideration of a new oral challenge protocol. J Allergy Clin Immunol Pract 2015;3:932.
28. White A, Bosso J, Stevenson D. The clinical dilemma of "silent desensitization" in aspirin-exacerbated respiratory disease. Allergy Asthma Proc 2013;34:378.
29. Lee J, Simon R, Sevenson D. Selection of aspirin dosages for aspirin desensitization treatment in patients with aspirin-exacerbated respiratory disease. J Allergy Clin Immunol 2007;119:157.
30. Rozsasi A, Polzehl D, Deutschle T, et al. Long-term treatment with aspirin desensitization: a prospective clinical trial comparing 100 and 300 mg aspirin daily. Allergy 2008;63:1228.

# Clinical Trials of Aspirin Treatment After Desensitization in Aspirin-Exacerbated Respiratory Disease

Marek L. Kowalski, MD, PhD[a],*, Aleksandra Wardzyńska, MD, PhD[a],
Joanna S. Makowska, MD, PhD[b]

## KEYWORDS

- Aspirin hypersensitivity • Aspirin desensitization
- Nonsteroidal anti-inflammatory drugs • NSAIDs-exacerbated respiratory disease
- Asthma • Chronic rhinosinusitis

## KEY POINTS

- Aspirin treatment after desensitization (ATAD) is an option in the management of patients with NSAID-exacerbated respiratory disease (N-ERD).
- Clinical efficacy of ATAD in patients with N-ERD has been documented in observational studies and in placebo-controlled double-blind trials.
- In most patients with N-ERD, ATAD is associated with a decrease in chronic rhinosinusitis symptoms and a reduction in nasal polyp recurrence.
- In a subset of patients with N-ERD, ATAD may result in decreased asthma symptoms and improved asthma control.
- Appropriate preventive measures may reduce the prevalence of adverse effects associated with ATAD.

## INTRODUCTION

Desensitization to aspirin was first reported in 1922 by the French physician Fernand Widal.[1] A 37-year-old woman with asthma, rhinitis, and nasal polyps had a convincing history of adverse reactions to small doses of aspirin and antipyrine manifesting with erythema, angioedema, and bronchospasm. Widal decided to begin a desensitization

[a] Department of Immunology, Rheumatology and Allergy, Healthy Ageing Research Center, Medical University of Łódź, 251 Pomorska Street, Łódź 92-213, Poland; [b] Department of Rheumatology, Medical University of Łódź, 30 Pieniny Street, Łódź 92-115, Poland
* Corresponding author.
E-mail address: Marek.Kowalski@csk.umed.lodz.pl

Immunol Allergy Clin N Am 36 (2016) 705–717
http://dx.doi.org/10.1016/j.iac.2016.06.007     immunology.theclinics.com
0889-8561/16/$ – see front matter © 2016 Elsevier Inc. All rights reserved.

procedure starting from a daily dose of 10 mg of acetylsalicylic acid (ASA) for 4 days. The dose was increased every 4 days (20 mg, 30 mg, 50 mg) until the patient eventually tolerated 600 mg of ASA. Following desensitization to ASA, a cross-tolerance of antipyrine was observed. However, the authors did not report if they continued treatment with aspirin after desensitization. Six decades later Stevenson and colleagues[2] described two aspirin-sensitive patients with asthma who were challenged with oral aspirin for investigative purposes. Following successful desensitization, the patients began taking 325 mg aspirin per day and after 6 and 8 months the aspirin dosage was increased to 650 mg per day. In both patients, during aspirin treatment, an improvement in symptoms of rhinitis and asthma was observed. In parallel, systemic corticosteroids had been reduced in one patient and discontinued in the other, while the lung function values were maintained unchanged.

Following the groundbreaking report by Stevenson and colleagues,[2] the efficacy of aspirin treatment after desensitization (ATAD) for the management of upper and lower respiratory disease in ASA-sensitive patients has been assessed in several studies and now is considered a valuable treatment modality in the management of some patients with nonsteroidal anti-inflammatory drug (NSAID)-exacerbated respiratory disease (N-ERD)[a].[3–5] Aspirin desensitization is a universal phenomenon, it can be achieved in almost all patients with N-ERD, and the tolerance can be maintained (in most patients) indefinitely with daily ASA.[6] Protocols for desensitization are usually extension of ASA-provocation protocols, but a "silent" desensitization (ie, without evoking adverse reaction) is possible if the procedure starts with a subthreshold dose of ASA and then the dose is slowly increased in appropriate intervals.[7,8]

More than 20 studies assessing clinical efficacy of treatment with aspirin on asthma and rhinosinusitis after desensitization have been published. In total, almost 1000 patients with N-ERD were desensitized and evaluated, however only four studies were placebo controlled. Clinical trials of ATAD varied in duration (2 weeks–6 years), dosing of ASA (100 mg–2600 mg) and clinical end points assessed (eg, symptoms; need for medication; exacerbation rate, polyp recurrence). Heterogeneity in trial design, ASA dosing, and duration of treatment make the pooling of data difficult, thus careful analysis of individual reports is a reasonable approach to evaluate the clinical efficacy and safety of this procedure. This article summarizes the data from noncontrolled, active-control, and placebo-controlled trials assessing clinical effectiveness and reporting on safety of treatment with ASA in desensitized patients with N-ERD.

## TRIALS OF ASPIRIN TREATMENT AFTER DESENSITIZATION NOT CONTROLLED WITH PLACEBO
### Effectiveness of Aspirin Treatment After Desensitization in Chronic Rhinosinusitis with Nasal Polyps

The effects of ATAD on the clinical course of chronic rhinosinusitis (CRS) with nasal polyposis were assessed in 18 studies published from 1983 to 2015, which included 798 patients. However, there is a significant variability in the trials design: in some the clinical outcomes in patients treated with aspirin were compared with parallel untreated or pharmacologically treated groups; in others, no control groups were included.

---

[a] Because most NSAID-induced hypersensitivity reactions are evoked by compounds other than aspirin, it has been proposed that it is more appropriate to use the term "NSAIDs" to replace "aspirin" in definitions of particular subtypes of aspirin hypersensitivity.[3] Accordingly, aspirin-exacerbated respiratory disease (AERD) could be substituted by NSAID-exacerbated respiratory disease (N-ERD).

All studies documented overall reduction of nasal symptoms (in most studies nasal congestion was the leading symptom that improved), and the percentage of patients reporting improvement varied from 33% in one relatively small study of Naejie and colleagues[9] to the average 66% in most studies and reaching even more than 90% in other studies.[10–12]

The effect of ATAD on anosmia was assessed by symptom score in 12 studies and all studies reported an overall improvement. In one study the sense of smell was assessed by an objective smell test and a significant improvement was observed after 1 and 3 months of treatment (mean four-fold increase in the smell test score).[13] In most patients whose nasal symptoms improved following treatment with ASA, a reduction of concomitant medications (intranasal corticosteroids) dose was possible.[11,14,15]

In some studies, objective parameters of nasal congestion also were assessed. Rozsasi and colleagues[16] demonstrated an improvement in rhinomanometric values after 12 months of treatment with 300 mg, but not after 100 mg of daily ASA. Makowska and colleagues[13] observed a significant (mean, 48%) improvement in nasal peak flow as early as 4 weeks after treatment with 600 mg of ASA.

Recurrent exacerbations of sinus disease related to upper airway infections have been considered as the major cause of morbidity in patients with CRS. In a retrospective observational study including 35 patients with N-ERD treated with aspirin and 42 patients with N-ERD avoiding NSAIDs, Sweet and colleagues[10] documented that the number of sinus infections were significantly reduced following ASA treatment. Several other studies reported fewer number of acute rhinosinusitis incidents (flares) corresponding to sinus infections, during treatment with ASA.[11,14,15,17]

Rhinonasal pathology in patients with N-ERD is characterized by chronic eosinophilic pansinusitis with mucosal hypertrophy manifesting as nasal polyposis. A high recurrence rate of nasal polyposis following standard nasal surgery or functional endoscopic sinus surgery (FESS) is a typical feature of N-ERD. In most studies in which polyp size was assessed by endoscopy or rhinofiberoscopy a significant reduction in polyp size was observed during ASA treatment.[12,16]

Most studies documented that ATAD inhibits regrowth of nasal polyps, decreasing the recurrence rate and/or delaying the time to the revision surgery.[10,11,14–18] Sweet and colleagues[10] and Stevenson and colleagues[17] in observational studies documented that 1300 mg of ASA daily may effectively decrease the need for sinus operations (eg, from one every 3 years to one in 9 years as reported by Stevenson and colleagues[17]).

More recently, Havel and colleagues[19] followed up two groups of patients with N-ERD undergoing FESS: one group was desensitized and treated with 500 mg of ASA and the second was treated with intranasal corticosteroids. Patients were followed at 1 year and then at long-term follow-up (from 18 to 84 months; mean, 36 months). Patients on ASA, in addition to significant improvement in all nasal symptoms (which included smell), had significantly fewer polyps and lower recurrence assessed by endoscopy when compared with control patients at the 1 year and the long-term follow-up. Furthermore, during long-term observation none of 56 aspirin-treated patients required further nasal surgery, whereas in the control group 7 out of 33 patients underwent sinus surgery, and 16 received a burst of oral corticosteroids to improve sinonasal symptoms. This study suggests that ATAD may be particularly effective in prevention of nasal polyps recurrence when patients are desensitized directly (within 1 month) following sinus surgery. Rozsasi and colleagues[16] in a small group of patients with N-ERD documented that even treatment with a daily dose of aspirin of 300 mg may prevent polyp recurrence. In their study no patient (n = 7) receiving 300 mg of aspirin during 18 months showed recurrent nasal polyps on endoscopic examination as compared with all (n = 7) patients receiving 100 mg of aspirin after desensitization. In one study[12] although ATAD resulted in symptomatic improvement, polyp size remained stable up to 30 months after desensitization as compared with postoperative evaluation, although no patient required additional sinus surgery during the follow-up period.

In the only study that assessed changes in sinonasal mucosal thickness using nuclear magnetic resonance, clinical improvements observed after 3 months of treatment with 650 mg of aspirin were not accompanied by any change in the thickness score, suggesting the lack of correlation between subjective and objective outcomes of ATAD.[13]

The effect of ATAD on quality of life related to CRS has been assessed in two studies. Havel and colleagues[19] reported a significant improvement in quality of life at 1 year and at long-term follow-up (minimum 18 months) in FESS patients treated with 500 mg of aspirin but not in a parallel group of patients on intranasal corticosteroids. In a recent study, a significant improvement in the quality of life related to CRS was reported as early as after 1 month of treatment with 650 mg of aspirin.[13]

Clinical benefit has been observed as early as 1 month after initiation of treatment[13,14,20] and could be maintained as long as the treatment lasted; even up to 5 to 7 years.[10,15,16,18] The effective maintenance dose of aspirin varied from 300 to 2600 mg daily, and no clear dose-related effects of aspirin have been demonstrated. Lee and colleagues[11] documented the clinical equivalence of 650 mg versus 1300 mg daily maintenance dose of aspirin with respect to number of sinus infections and sinus surgeries after 1 year of treatment. Simon and colleagues[21] recommend starting treatment after desensitization with 650 mg twice daily, and then, after 1 month, if effective control of symptoms is observed the dose can be reduced by half. However, clinical effectiveness of lower doses of ASA (300 mg) also has been documented,[14,16] thus it is reasonable to tailor the maintenance dose of aspirin in individual patients to balance clinical effectiveness with potential risk of adverse symptoms (gastrointestinal [GI] symptoms, bleeding).[11]

In a systematic review of the literature on ATAD for nasal polyposis in patients with N-ERD, Xu and colleagues[22] analyzed nine studies of oral and two of intranasal treatment with aspirin published between 1995 and 2013. They were able to assign level 2 evidence to nine cohort studies of oral ATAD, seven of which were considered to have a satisfactory quality score. Although overall a significant improvement in symptom scores, decrease in corticosteroid use, and decrease in revision surgery was reported in most studies, they concluded that "heterogeneity between trials prevents pooling of data and a clear-cut answer remains lacking."

The overall evidence from these uncontrolled studies, although clinically convincing, is of low quality because of methodologic limitations: lack of patient randomization to ASA and control (usually active treatment) groups, variability in ASA dosing and duration of treatment, and paucity of reported objective parameters. Furthermore, concomitant pharmacologic treatment in aspirin and control groups has not been consistently reported and lack of blinding and placebo control does not allow the exclusion of reporting bias.

### Intranasal Desensitization and Treatment with Aspirin

Local tolerance to aspirin can be achieved following repeated intranasal application of lysine aspirin and prolonged local treatment has been shown to alleviate the upper airway symptoms and reduce recurrence rates for polyposis in patients with N-ERD.[23,24] However, the beneficial effects of intranasal aspirin were not confirmed in a double-blind placebo-controlled trial.[25] More recently, Howe and colleagues[26] followed up 105 patients with N-ERD treated with self-administered intranasal lysine aspirin for 3 months (first assessment; n = 60 patients) or 12 months (second assessment; n = 27). A significant improvement in nasal peak flow, olfaction, and nasal nitric oxide levels was observed at both time points. Interestingly, in a subgroup of patients (n = 20) several asthma outcomes also improved (decrease in emergency visits, hospitalization, and oral steroid use).

### Effects of Aspirin Treatment After Desensitization on Bronchial Asthma Outcomes

In most studies discussed previously that assessed CRS outcomes following ATAD, the effects of aspirin on bronchial asthma outcomes were also analyzed. However, interpretation of the effect of ATAD on asthma is more difficult because improvements in some outcomes may reflect effects of aspirin on upper and lower respiratory diseases (eg, decrease in maintenance dose of systemic corticosteroids or number of unscheduled office visits). In two long-term studies from the same center (Scripps Clinic, La Jolla, CA) patients were treated with daily aspirin for a minimum of 1 and up to 6 years. Along with improvement in CRS symptoms, a beneficial effect on asthma was observed.[10,14] In most patients (more than 90%), the maintenance doses of oral and inhaled corticosteroids were reduced and a decrease in number of emergency room visits and hospitalizations was observed when compared with the control group. However, in another study of Stevenson and colleagues[17] treatment with 1300 mg of aspirin daily for a mean of 3.3 years (range, 1–6 years) resulted in decreased numbers of asthma hospitalizations per year, but did not reduce the number of emergency visits for asthma or use of inhaled corticosteroids. The beneficial effect of aspirin on asthma exacerbation rate, number of hospitalizations, emergency room visits, or corticosteroid courses was also observed following 1 year of treatment with a small dose of aspirin (300 mg/daily).[15] The effects of ATAD on respiratory function are less consistent: in three studies improvement of pulmonary function was observed,[16,27–30] whereas in another three the forced expiratory volume in 1 second value did not change significantly.[9,15,20]

The overall effect of aspirin on asthma seems to be less favorable as compared with the effect on the course of CRS: out of 15 uncontrolled studies evaluating the effect of ASA treatment on asthma, nine documented overall significant improvement in various asthma outcomes.[9–11,14–17,28,29] In two studies, only half of patients reported any beneficial effects.[20,30] Conversely, in one long-term study with 500 mg of aspirin no improvement in asthma symptoms was reported,[19] whereas in another study, most patients experienced asthma deterioration.[31]

In conclusion, these uncontrolled studies (which usually had a reference, parallel group on standard asthma therapy) reported improvement in asthma symptoms in variable proportion of patients, but predictive factors for asthma improvement with ATAD have not been identified. In the study of Forster-Ruhrmann and colleagues[27] the clinical effects of ATAD on asthma control and respiratory function parameters were observed during 18 months of treatment, but only in the group of patients with uncontrolled asthma, suggesting that people with severe asthma may profit more from ATAD.

## DOUBLE-BLIND PLACEBO-CONTROLLED TRIALS OF ASPIRIN TREATMENT AFTER DESENSITIZATION

By January 2016, four double-blind placebo-controlled trials of ATAD have been published, involving a total of 163 patients with N-ERD from which 103 completed the trial period (**Table 1**).[32–35]

**Table 1**
Double-blind placebo-controlled trials of aspirin treatment after desensitization in patients with N-ERD

| Author | # of Patients Evaluated | ASA Maintenance Dose | Duration of Treatment | Effect of ATAD on Rhinosinusitis | Effect of ATAD on Asthma |
|---|---|---|---|---|---|
| Stevenson et al,[32] 1984 | 25 (both ASA and placebo in a crossover study) | 325–1300 mg and 2600 mg | 3 mo | Lower total nasal symptom score; improvement in smell | No change in asthma symptom scores or prednisone maintenance doses |
| Fruth et al,[34] 2013 | ASA, 18; Placebo, 13 | 100 mg | 36 mo | Lower nasal symptom score, including improvement in smell; tendency for decreased relapse rate of nasal polyps | Not assessed |
| Świerczyńska et al,[33] 2014 | N-ERD: ASA, 8; Placebo, 7 Aspirin tolerant: ASA, 5; Placebo, 8 | 624 mg | 6 mo | Lower nasal symptom score, no improvement in sinus involvement | Decrease in dose of ICS; improved asthma control No change in asthma symptom scores or FEV$_1$ |
| Esmaeilzadeh et al,[35] 2015 | ASA, 18; Placebo, 16 | 1300 mg | 6 mo | Lower nasal symptom score, improvement in sinus involvement | Lower asthma symptom scores, improvement in FEV$_1$ |

*Abbreviations:* FEV$_1$, forced expiratory volume in 1 second; ICS, inhaled corticosteroids.

In the first double-blind placebo-controlled study with a crossover design published by Stevenson and colleagues[32] patients with N-ERD received 325 mg, 1300 mg, or 2600 mg of ASA or placebo for 3 months. During a 3-month treatment with aspirin following desensitization, patients demonstrated a significant improvement in the combined nasal symptom score and reduced dosing of intranasal beclomethasone. Individual nasal symptoms, such as nasal congestion and sinus pain, were also reduced, but runny nose, sense of smell, or postnasal discharge did not improve as compared with the placebo period. The overall asthma symptom scores or prednisone maintenance doses used for asthma control were not significantly reduced, and respiratory function remained similar during both treatment periods. Thus, although in this study the beneficial effect of ASA on CRS symptoms was clearly documented, no effect on asthma symptoms was demonstrated. For upper airway symptoms, no significant dose-response relationship was noticed, although there was a tendency toward better efficacy of higher doses of ASA.

Fruth and colleagues[34] assessed only CRS outcomes in patients with N-ERD treated with ASA or placebo, with a primary outcome defined as nasal polyps relapse after 36 months of treatment. Following sinus surgery, patients were desensitized and treated with a low dose of aspirin (100 mg daily) or were assigned to receive placebo. Because of a very high dropout rate (66%) only 18 patients with active treatment and 13 of the placebo group were evaluated. The overall symptoms score and intensity of nasal/paranasal complaints were significantly lower in the ASA group and the quality of life and quality of life related to nasal problems were better in the active treatment group. ASA-treated patients demonstrated a significantly more pronounced improvement in their sense of smell after 36 months. Nasal polyp recurrence after 3 years of treatment was observed in 62% of patients on placebo and in 28% of patients receiving ASA for 3 years; however, the difference was not statistically significant. Although the power of this study is limited by a very high dropout rate, it demonstrated a potential for effective treatment with a low dose of aspirin after desensitization, and an acute need for studies assessing for a dose-response in ATAD.

Świerczyńska-Krępa and colleagues[33] published a double-blind placebo-controlled study, including for the first time both patients with N-ERD and aspirin-tolerant subjects with asthma to receive, in a double-blind fashion, placebo or 624 mg of ASA for 6 months. Overall nasal symptom scores (SNOT20), sneezing, nasal blockage, and sneezing decreased, and smell scores were improved during ASA treatment as compared with baseline only in patients with N-ERD. However, the computed tomography (CT) scores were similar to those at baseline and did not parallel clinical improvement. Asthma control scores after 6 month of treatment were improved and the doses of inhaled corticosteroids were reduced in patients with N-ERD treated with ASA as compared with the N-ERD group receiving placebo. However, asthma symptoms, use of rescue medications, or respiratory function parameters (forced expiratory volume in 1 second and peak expiratory flow rate values) did not change throughout the 6-month chronic ASA course. This study, despite including a low number of patients, demonstrated for the first time that treatment with ASA may be effective only in patients hypersensitive to NSAIDs, but not in NSAID-tolerant patients with rhinosinusitis and asthma.

A recently published study[35] evaluated 18 patients with N-ERD receiving 625 mg of aspirin twice daily and 16 patients receiving placebo for 6 months. Although no significant change in clinical outcomes was observed at 1 month, after 6 months of treatment patients in the active arm had significantly improved symptom and medication scores and higher spirometric values compared with baseline and with the placebo group. The primary outcome of the study (quality of life) significantly improved only in the ASA-treated group and was better compared with the group receiving placebo. Sinus involvement assessed on CT scans with the Lund-Mackay score was significantly reduced (by mean 26%) after 6 months of active treatment; however, it is noted that patients in the placebo arm had lower CT score values at baseline.

These double-blind placebo-controlled trials, although differing in design, dose of ASA, and duration of treatment, consistently confirm the beneficial effects of ATAD on most CRS outcomes in patients with N-ERD, whereas the effects on asthma outcomes seem to be less consistent.

## ADVERSE EFFECTS AND EARLY DISCONTINUATION OF ACETYLSALICYLIC ACID TREATMENT AFTER DESENSITIZATION

Chronic treatment with ASA after desensitization is associated with adverse effects and the incidence of adverse symptoms related to ASA in various studies ranged from 0% to 34%, without difference between placebo-controlled trials (range, 0% to 33%) and noncontrolled studies (0%–34%) (**Table 2**). The most prevalent adverse effects were GI symptoms that are usually mild: dyspepsia, stomach pain, gastric upset or irritation. GI bleeding has been reported in a few patients, although in no case was bleeding associated with serious complications.[11,14,35] GI symptoms have been the most common reason for discontinuation of ASA therapy. Other adverse effects reported incidentally during ATAD include skin symptoms (rash, urticaria),[14,34,35] epistaxis or ecchymosis,[11,15] worsening of asthma,[11,18] and increase in nasal symptoms.[14]

It is not clear if the prevalence of adverse reactions during treatment with ASA after desensitization is dose related. However, in studies with low maintenance ASA doses (up to 500 mg/daily) the incidence GI symptoms (0%–8%) and the discontinuation rate from ASA side effects (range, 0%–10%) seemed to be lower than in trials with high (>650 mg/day) ASA doses (range, 0%–34% and 0%–34% for GI symptoms and dropouts, respectively) (see **Table 2**). However, comparing the incidence of side effects between studies using various dosing of aspirin is difficult because of differences in methodology, which include various inclusion criteria (eg, exclusion of subjects with any GI diseases or symptoms) or not reporting concomitant treatment with GI prophylaxis. Lee and colleagues,[11] who compared the efficacy of two different doses of ASA, observed similar frequency of side effects caused by aspirin intake in patients maintained on 1300 mg or 650 mg of aspirin per day. Similarly, in a study comparing treatment with low doses of ASA (100 mg/day vs 300 mg/day) there were no significant differences in the prevalence of adverse effects between those two doses.[16]

Recently, Makowska and colleagues[13] reported a significant decrease in urinary creatinine levels after 1 month of treatment with 650 mg in all desensitized patients with N-ERD. Urinary creatinine was further decreased after 2 and 3 months of treatment with ASA (**Fig. 1**), although it was not accompanied by any changes in serum creatinine, suggesting that renal function was not significantly affected. Similar effects of NSAIDs (cyclooxygenase-1 and -2 inhibitors) on renal function have been reported earlier in 1% to 5% of patients treated with NSAIDs.[36] Production of prostaglandin $E_2$ by renal epithelium is important for maintaining renal blood flow and the inhibition by NSAIDs of prostaglandin $E_2$ production may result in decreased renal filtration. One can speculate that in patients with N-ERD who may be more susceptible to cyclooxygenase inhibition by NSAIDs, ASA treatment may have an even more pronounced effect on prostaglandin $E_2$ production in renal epithelium and on renal function compared with ASA-tolerant subjects. Future studies are necessary to clarify the importance of these findings to the safety of treatment with ASA in patients with N-ERD.

**Table 2**
Early discontinuation of aspirin treatment after desensitization

| Author | ASA Maintenance Dose | Discontinuation Rate (%) | Reasons for Discontinuation (%) |
|---|---|---|---|
| Sweet et al,[10] 1990 | 325–2600 mg | 16/35 (45.7) | Related to ASA: 12/35 (34); GI intolerance, 12 |
| Stevenson et al,[17] 1996 | 1300 mg | 13/78 (16.7) | • Related to ASA: 9/75 (11.5); gastric pain, 7; gastric, bleeding, 2<br>• Unrelated to ASA: 4 |
| Gosepath et al,[28] 2001 | 100 mg | 0/30 | 0 |
| Berges-Gimeno et al,[29] 2003 | 1300 mg | 0/38 | 0 |
| Berges-Gimeno et al,[14] 2003 | 1300 mg | 46/172 (26.7) | • Related to ASA: 24/172 (18.8); gastric pain, 14; gastric bleeding, 2; nose, ear bleeding, 2; urticaria, 6<br>• Unrelated to ASA: 22 |
| Lee et al,[11] 2007 | 650 mg | 18/70 (25.7) | • Related to ASA: 14/70 (20); dyspepsia, 9; urticaria, 3; asthma worsening, 1; ecchymosis, 1; tinnitus, 1<br>• Unrelated to ASA: 2 |
|  | 1300 mg | 14/67 (20.9) | • Related to ASA: 10/67 (14.9); dyspepsia, 3; angioedema, 1; bleeding, 2; asthma, 3; ecchymosis, 1<br>• Unrelated to ASA: 4 |
| Rozsasi et al,[16] 2008 | 300 mg | 2/39 (5.1) | Related to ASA: 2/39 (5.1); GI intolerance, 2 |
| Comert et al,[15] 2013 | 300 mg | 18/40 (45) | • Related to ASA: 4/40 (10); GI side effects, 3; ecchymosis, 1<br>• Unrelated to ASA: 14 |
| Havel et al,[19] 2013 | 500 mg | 9/65 (13.8) | 0 |
| Cho et al,[12] 2014 | ? | 7/28 (25) | • Related to ASA: 1/28 (3.6); GI side effects, 1<br>• Unrelated to ASA: 6 |
| Ibrahim et al,[40] 2014 | 650–1300 mg | 29/111 (26.1) | • Related to ASA: 26/111 (23.4); GI upset, 23; easy bruising, 3<br>• Unrelated to ASA: 3 |
| Spies et al,[18] 2016 | 1300 mg for 6 mo then decreases | 8/16 (50) | • Related to ASA: 3/16 (18.8); asthma worsening, 3<br>• Unrelated to ASA: 5 |
| Placebo-controlled |  |  |  |
| Stevenson et al,[32] 1984 | 325–1300 mg and 2600 mg | 13/25 (52) | • Related to ASA: 2/25 (8); GI pain, 2<br>• Unrelated to ASA: 11 |
| Fruth et al,[34] 2013 | 100 mg | 18/36 (50) in active arm | Unrelated to ASA: 18 |
| Świerczyńska et al,[33] 2014 | 624 | 4/12 (33) in active AIA arm, 1/8 (12.5) in active ATA arm | • Related to ASA: 4/12 (33) in active aspirin induced asthma arm; dyspepsia, 4 (1 dyspepsia + rash); 1/8 (12.5) in active aspirin tolerant asthma arm; dyspepsia, 1<br>• Unrelated to ASA: 11 |
| Esmaeilzadeh et al,[35] 2015 | 1300 mg | 2/18 (11.1) in active arm | Related to ASA: 2/18 (11.1) in active arm; GI bleeding, 1; skin rash, 1 |

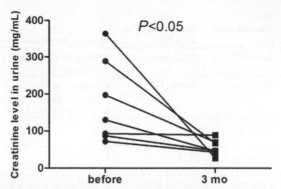

**Fig. 1.** Effects of aspirin treatment on urinary creatinine levels before and 3 months after desensitization. (*From* Makowska JS, Olszewska-Ziaber A, Bieńkiewicz B, et al. Clinical benefits of aspirin desensitization in patients with NSAID-Exacerbated Respiratory Disease (NERD) are not related to urinary eicosanoid release, and are accompanied with decreased urine creatinine. Allergy Asthma Proc 2016;37(3):220; with permission.)

Overall, 37% (range, 0%–52%) of patients treated with ATAD dropped out from trials because of reasons related and nonrelated directly to treatment-induced side effects: GI symptom, bleeding, skin rash, asthma exacerbations, increased nasal symptoms, and lack of interest to continue. The highest dropout rate was reported by Fruth and colleagues,[34] but despite a long duration of treatment none of the patients actually dropped out because of side effects of aspirin (100 mg of daily ASA in this study).

## MEASURES TO IMPROVE GASTRIC SAFETY OF ASPIRIN TREATMENT AFTER DESENSITIZATION

The use of GI prophylaxis in patients on maintenance doses of ASA seems to prevent development of GI symptoms during ATAD. In a study by Spies and colleagues[18] in which all patients received proton pump inhibitors or $H_2$ blockers there was no single case of ASA-therapy discontinuation because of GI symptoms, despite high maintenance doses of aspirin (1300 mg/day). Although there is a concern that prolonged treatment with proton pump inhibitors may be associated with side effects,[37] recent studies showed that in cardiovascular patients treated with cardioprotective doses of ASA for long periods, proton pump inhibitors reduced the risk of GI bleeding.[38] Because the presence of *Helicobacter pylori* is a known risk factor for the GI side effects of NSAIDs, it has been suggested that eradication of *H pylori* should be considered before desensitization.[39]

## SUMMARY AND FUTURE CONSIDERATIONS

The clinical efficacy of ATAD in patients with N-ERD has been documented in observational studies and in double-blind placebo-controlled trials. It seems to be particularly effective and should be recommended in patients with N-ERD with refractory CRS with nasal polyps requiring either frequent systemic corticosteroid bursts or repeated revision sinus surgeries. In parallel with the improvement in CRS outcomes, ATAD may alleviate asthma symptoms and improve asthma control in some patients, although usually this is not associated with improvement in pulmonary function parameters.

Chronic treatment with ASA after desensitization is associated with adverse reactions, which may result in early discontinuation of treatment in about one-third of treated patients. Specific preventive measures, including the use of GI prophylaxis, should be implemented in desensitized patients during chronic treatment with ASA. There is no general agreement with regard to the optimal maintenance dose or duration of treatment with ASA after desensitization, thus further studies are necessary to offer clear guidelines to clinicians. Further investigations to understand the mechanisms that lead to improvements in CRS and asthma during ATAD should allow the identification of subsets of patients with N-ERD, who would benefit most from this treatment modality.

## REFERENCES

1. Widal F, Abrami P, Lermoyez J. Anaphylaxie et idiosyncrasie. La Press Medicale 1922;30:189–93.
2. Stevenson DD, Simon RA, Mathison DA. Aspirin-sensitive asthma: tolerance to aspirin after positive oral aspirin challenges. J Allergy Clin Immunol 1980;66:82–8.
3. Kowalski ML, Asero R, Bavbek S, et al. Classification and practical approach to the diagnosis and management of hypersensitivity to nonsteroidal anti-inflammatory drugs. Allergy 2013;68:1219–32.
4. White AA, Stevenson DD. Aspirin desensitization in aspirin-exacerbated respiratory disease. Immunol Allergy Clin North Am 2013;33:211–22.
5. Simon RA, Dazy KM, Waldram JD. Update on aspirin desensitization for chronic rhinosinusitis with polyps in aspirin-exacerbated respiratory disease (AERD). Curr Allergy Asthma Rep 2015;15:508.
6. Stevenson DD. Aspirin sensitivity and desensitization for asthma and sinusitis. Curr Allergy Asthma Rep 2009;9:155–63.
7. Szmidt M, Grzelewska-Rzymowska I, Kowalski ML, et al. Tolerance to acetylsalicylic acid (ASA) induced in ASA-sensitive asthmatics does not depend on initial adverse reaction. Allergy 1987;42:182–5.
8. White AA, Bosso JV, Stevenson DD. The clinical dilemma of "silent desensitization" in aspirin-exacerbated respiratory disease. Allergy Asthma Proc 2013;34:378–82.
9. Naeije N, Bracamonte M, Michel O, et al. Effects of chronic aspirin ingestion in aspirin-intolerant asthmatic patients. Ann Allergy 1984;53:262–4.
10. Sweet JM, Stevenson DD, Simon RA, et al. Long-term effects of aspirin desensitization–treatment for aspirin-sensitive rhinosinusitis-asthma. J Allergy Clin Immunol 1990;85:59–65.
11. Lee JY, Simon RA, Stevenson DD. Selection of aspirin dosages for aspirin desensitization treatment in patients with aspirin-exacerbated respiratory disease. J Allergy Clin Immunol 2007;119:157–64.
12. Cho KS, Soudry E, Psaltis AJ, et al. Long-term sinonasal outcomes of aspirin desensitization in aspirin exacerbated respiratory disease. Otolaryngol Head Neck Surg 2014;151:575–81.
13. Makowska JS, Olszewska-Ziaber A, Bieńkiewicz B, et al. Clinical benefits of aspirin desensitization in patients with NSAID-Exacerbated Respiratory Disease (NERD) are not related to urinary eicosanoid release, and are accompanied with decreased urine creatinine. Allergy Asthma Proc 2016;37(3):216–24.
14. Berges-Gimeno MP, Simon RA, Stevenson DD. Long-term treatment with aspirin desensitization in asthmatic patients with aspirin-exacerbated respiratory disease. J Allergy Clin Immunol 2003;111:180–6.

15. Comert S, Celebioglu E, Yucel T, et al. Aspirin 300 mg/day is effective for treating aspirin-exacerbated respiratory disease. Allergy 2013;68:1443–51.

16. Rozsasi A, Polzehl D, Deutschle T, et al. Long-term treatment with aspirin desensitization: a prospective clinical trial comparing 100 and 300 mg aspirin daily. Allergy 2008;63:1228–34.

17. Stevenson DD, Hankammer MA, Mathison DA, et al. Aspirin desensitization treatment of aspirin-sensitive patients with rhinosinusitis-asthma: long-term outcomes. J Allergy Clin Immunol 1996;98:751–8.

18. Spies JW, Valera FP, Cordeiro DL, et al. The role of aspirin desensitization in patients with aspirin-exacerbated respiratory disease (AERD). Braz J Otorhinolaryngol 2016;82(3):263–8.

19. Havel M, Ertl L, Braunschweig F, et al. Sinonasal outcome under aspirin desensitization following functional endoscopic sinus surgery in patients with aspirin triad. Eur Arch Otorhinolaryngol 2013;270:571–8.

20. Kowalski ML, Grzelewska-Rzymowska I, Szmidt M, et al. Clinical efficacy of aspirin in "desensitized" aspirin-sensitive asthmatics. Eur J Respir Dis 1986;69: 219–25.

21. Simon RA, Dazy KM, Waldram JD. Aspirin-exacerbated respiratory disease: characteristics and management strategies. Expert Rev Clin Immunol 2015;11: 805–17.

22. Xu JJ, Sowerby L, Rotenberg BW. Aspirin desensitization for aspirin-exacerbated respiratory disease (Samter's Triad): a systematic review of the literature. Int Forum Allergy Rhinol 2013;3:915–20.

23. Patriarca G, Bellioni P, Nucera E, et al. Intranasal treatment with lysine acetylsalicylate in patients with nasal polyposis. Ann Allergy 1991;67:588–92.

24. Ogata N, Darby Y, Scadding G. Intranasal lysine-aspirin administration decreases polyp volume in patients with aspirin-intolerant asthma. J Laryngol Otol 2007;121:1156–60.

25. Parikh AA, Scadding GK. Intranasal lysine-aspirin in aspirin-sensitive nasal polyposis: a controlled trial. Laryngoscope 2005;115:1385–90.

26. Howe R, Mirakian RM, Pillai P, et al. Audit of nasal lysine aspirin therapy in recalcitrant aspirin exacerbated respiratory disease. World Allergy Organ J 2014;7:18.

27. Förster-Ruhrmann U, Zappe SM, Szczepek AJ, et al. Long-term clinical effects of aspirin-desensitization therapy among patients with poorly controlled asthma and non-steroidal anti-inflammatory drug hypersensitivity: an exploratory study. Rev Port Pneumol (2006) 2015. [Epub ahead of print].

28. Gosepath J, Schaefer D, Amedeee RG, et al. Individual monitoring of aspirin desensitization. Arch Otolaryngol Head Neck Surg 2001;127:316–21.

29. Berges-Gimeno MP, Simon RA, Stevenson DD. Early effects of aspirin desensitization treatment in asthmatic patients with aspirin-exacerbated respiratory disease. Ann Allergy Asthma Immunol 2003;90:338–41.

30. Chiu JT. Improvement in aspirin-sensitive asthmatic subjects after rapid aspirin desensitization and aspirin maintenance (ADAM) treatment. J Allergy Clin Immunol 1983;71:560–7.

31. Dor PJ, Vervloet D, Baldocchi G, et al. Aspirin intolerance and asthma induction of a tolerance and long-term monitoring. Clin Allergy 1985;15:37–42.

32. Stevenson DD, Pleskow WW, Simon RA, et al. Aspirin-sensitive rhinosinusitis asthma: a double-blind crossover study of treatment with aspirin. J Allergy Clin Immunol 1984;73:500–7.

33. Świerczyńska-Krępa M, Sanak M, Bochenek G, et al. Aspirin desensitization in patients with aspirin-induced and aspirin-tolerant asthma: a double-blind study. J Allergy Clin Immunol 2014;134:883–90.
34. Fruth K, Pogorzelski B, Schmidtmann I, et al. Low-dose aspirin desensitization in individuals with aspirin-exacerbated respiratory disease. Allergy 2013;68: 659–65.
35. Esmaeilzadeh H, Nabavi M, Aryan Z, et al. Aspirin desensitization for patients with aspirin-exacerbated respiratory disease: a randomized double-blind placebo-controlled trial. Clin Immunol 2015;160:349–57.
36. Segal R, Lubart E, Leibovitz A, et al. Early and late effects of low-dose aspirin on renal function in elderly patients. Am J Med 2003;115:462–6.
37. White AA, Stevenson DD. Side effects from daily aspirin treatment in patients with AERD: identification and management. Allergy Asthma Proc 2011;32:333–4.
38. Schjerning Olsen AM, Lindhardsen J, Gislason GH, et al. Impact of proton pump inhibitor treatment on gastrointestinal bleeding associated with non-steroidal anti-inflammatory drug use among post-myocardial infarction patients taking antithrombotics: nationwide study. BMJ 2015;351:h5096.
39. Makowska J, Makowski M, Kowalski ML. NSAIDs hypersensitivity: when and how to desensitize? Curr Treat Options Allergy 2015;2:124–40.
40. Ibrahim C, Singh K, Tsai G, et al. A retrospective study of the clinical benefit from acetylsalicylic acid desensitization in patients with nasal polyposis and asthma. Allergy Asthma Clin Immunol 2014;10:64.

# Eosinophils and Mast Cells in Aspirin-Exacerbated Respiratory Disease

 CrossMark

John W. Steinke, PhD[a], Spencer C. Payne, MD[b,c], Larry Borish, MD[a,d],*

## KEYWORDS

- Eosinophil • Mast cell • Leukotriene • Cyclooxygenase • Prostaglandin
- Aspirin-exacerbated respiratory disease • Arachidonic acid

## KEY POINTS

- Aspirin-exacerbated respiratory disease (AERD) is a disease of overproduction and hyper-responsiveness to lipid mediators.
- Mast cells and eosinophils are key drivers of AERD pathogenesis through production of proinflammatory mediators following aspirin stimulation.
- Because of their involvement, therapies that target mast cells and eosinophils may be useful in providing clinical benefit in AERD.

## INTRODUCTION

In 1968, the term Samter triad was coined and was defined by the presence of nasal polyps, aspirin sensitivity, and asthma[1]; however this disease is now referred to as aspirin-exacerbated respiratory disease (AERD) because asthma is not always present despite reactions to aspirin. AERD comprises as many as 7% of adult-onset asthmatics and up to 12% to 14% of adult asthmatics with severe asthma.[2,3] This disorder is characterized by the unique intolerance to aspirin and other nonselective cyclooxygenase (COX) inhibitors.[4–6] Other characteristics include hypereosinophilia, both in the circulation and in the tissue; a tendency to develop de novo in adulthood[5,7,8]; and often an absence of identifiable atopy.[5,7] Sinusitis is present in this disorder,

Supported by NIH grants R01AI057438, R56AI120055, and U01AI100799.

[a] Department of Medicine, Asthma and Allergic Disease Center, Carter Center for Immunology Research, University of Virginia Health System, 409 Lane Rd, Charlottesville, VA 22908, USA; [b] Department of Medicine, University of Virginia Health System, 409 Lane Rd, Charlottesville, VA 22908, USA; [c] Department of Otolaryngology – Head and Neck Surgery, University of Virginia Health System, 409 Lane Rd, Charlottesville, VA 22908, USA; [d] Department of Microbiology, Asthma and Allergic Disease Center, Carter Center for Immunology Research, University of Virginia Health System, 409 Lane Rd, Charlottesville, VA 22908, USA
* Corresponding author. Asthma and Allergic Disease Center, University of Virginia Health System, Box 801355, Charlottesville, VA 22908.
E-mail address: lb4m@virginia.edu

Immunol Allergy Clin N Am 36 (2016) 719–734
http://dx.doi.org/10.1016/j.iac.2016.06.008
0889-8561/16/$ – see front matter © 2016 Elsevier Inc. All rights reserved.
immunology.theclinics.com

the degree of which is often severe, and this is associated with complete or near-complete opacification of the sinus cavity.[8] Although not a requirement, when asthma is present it often progresses in severity and is associated with aggressive airway remodeling.[9]

During aspirin reactions, many mediators are released, including cysteinyl leukotrienes (CysLTs), tryptase, eosinophil cationic protein (ECP), and prostaglandin $D_2$ ($PGD_2$), suggesting both mast cell and eosinophil activation.[10–12] Recently, aspirin was shown to directly activate both of these cell types ex vivo potentiating mediator release.[13] A predominant physiologic feature of AERD is the robust overproduction and overresponsiveness to CysLTs (inflammatory),[11,14] while at the same time there is underproduction and underresponsiveness to the antiinflammatory lipid mediator $PGE_2$.[15–17] These CysLTs have important proinflammatory and profibrotic effects that contribute to the asthma severity and to the extensive hyperplastic sinusitis and nasal polyposis.[8,18,19] In addition, conversely, the downregulation of $PGE_2$ pathways reduces the constraints that would normally act to attenuate these proinflammatory pathways.[20] This article focuses on the role that eosinophils and mast cells play in contributing to these cardinal features of AERD.

## EOSINOPHIL AND MAST CELL NUMBERS IN ASPIRIN-EXACERBATED RESPIRATORY DISEASE

Chronic sinusitis (CRS) is now recognized as a collection of disorders that result from inflammation of the sinuses and in many cases can be separated into different types based on the cellular infiltrate. One distinguishing feature in the nasal polyps that often form in association with chronic sinusitis is the presence or absence of eosinophils and among eosinophilic polyps a distinction can be made between AERD, allergic fungal sinusitis (AFS), and chronic hyperplastic eosinophilic sinusitis (CHES).[21,22] Within the eosinophilic polyps, AERD has more than twice the number of eosinophils in the polyp tissue than AFS or CHES, implicating them as important cells in the disease process.[22] Examination of bronchial biopsies from patients with AERD also revealed highly increased eosinophil numbers compared with aspirin-tolerant asthmatics and nonasthmatics.[23] These eosinophils were in an activated state, as shown by the presence of secretory ECP.[23]

The authors have reported lower numbers of mast cells in nasal polyps from eosinophilic sinus disease compared with healthy tissue by both toluidine blue and chloroacetate (chymase) staining, and there was no difference between aspirin-tolerant and AERD groups.[22] This finding contrasts with a previous report that found no difference in mast cell numbers in nasal polyps from AERD groups compared with allergic or nonallergic individuals via tryptase staining.[24] The differences in the results of these studies may reflect the use of different markers of mast cells (chymase vs tryptase) or the stratification of the groups, the study by Park and colleagues[24] not taking into account eosinophilic infiltration into the polyp tissue. Regardless, there do not seem to be more mast cells in nasal polyps in patients with AERD. However, this result may be erroneous, given the high expression of mast cell–derived mediators, and perhaps reflects the inability to stain for activated, granule-depleted mast cells (so-called phantom mast cells). Similarly, when the lungs have been examined, as with nasal polyposis (NP), smaller numbers of mast cells have been found in patients with AERD compared with nonasthmatic controls using immunohistochemistry to stain for tryptase-positive cells.[23] Another study examining the bronchial mucosa found increased numbers of tryptase-positive mast cells only in subjects with non–aspirin-sensitive asthma: again, patients with AERD and healthy controls paradoxically had similar numbers.[25]

## DEVELOPMENT OF EOSINOPHILS AND MAST CELLS

Eosinophils develop from pluripotent hematopoietic stem cells in bone marrow that initially differentiate into eosinophil/basophil progenitors or colony-forming units (Eo/ B CFU) (**Fig. 1**). Eo/B CFU are mononuclear cells that express CD34, CD35, and inter-leukin (IL)-5 receptors (CD125) that are capable of responding to appropriate cytokine signals, allowing differentiation into mature basophils and eosinophils.[26,27] Eo/B CFU are increased in numbers in both the blood and bone marrow of allergic patients and further increases in their numbers are observed following allergen exposure.[27] These progenitors are also observed in nasal polyp tissue.[28] Several transcription factors, including GATA-1, PU.1, and C/EBP, are induced in response to appropriate cytokine signals and become involved in the development of the eosinophil lineage and eosinophil-associated genes.[29–31] In vitro eosinophil differentiation experiments have shown that GATA-1 is the primary transcription factor responsible for this eosin-ophil lineage specification.[32]

Three cytokines, IL-3, IL-5, and granulocyte-macrophage colony-stimulating factor (GM-CSF) play the most important roles in the regulation of eosinophil development (see **Fig. 1**). The function of IL-3 is the broadest because it leads to the expansion of a variety of cell types, including monocytes, megakaryocytes, erythrocytes, baso-phils, neutrophils, and eosinophils.[26] GM-CSF acts in a similar fashion, albeit with more mature precursor cells, inducing the formation of macrophages, neutrophils, and eosinophils.[33] IL-5 is the cytokine responsible for selective terminal differentiation of eosinophils[34] and stimulates the release of eosinophils from the bone marrow into

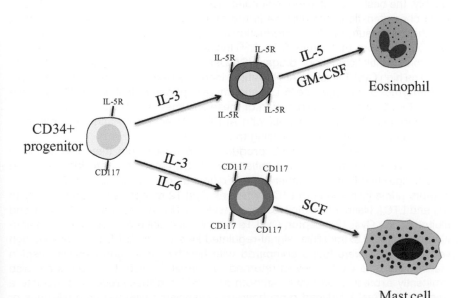

**Fig. 1.** Eosinophil and mast cell development from CD34 progenitor cells. Through the ac-tions of interleukin (IL)-3, IL-5, and granulocyte-macrophage colony-stimulating factor (GM-CSF), CD34 progenitor cells mature into eosinophils. Mast cells develop following stim-ulation with IL-3, IL-6, and stem cell factor (SCF) from CD34 progenitor cells.

peripheral circulation.[35] GM-CSF, IL-3, and the chemokines CCL11, CCL24, and CCL26 (eotaxins) are also involved in eosinophil homeostasis and play an important role on arrival of the eosinophil at a tissue location. In addition, an interferon gamma (IFN-γ)–induced transcription factor ICSBP (IFN consensus sequence binding protein) can also drive the differentiation of eosinophils.[36] Because IFN-γ is routinely present in allergic inflammation and, in our studies, was particularly upregulated in AERD,[37] this led us to speculate on the role of IFN-γ being able to contribute to eosinophilia. Using an in vitro model with CD34[+] hematopoietic progenitors, the authors showed the capacity of IFN-γ, acting in synergy with IL-5, to promote the survival and differentiation of mature bilobed, CCR3-expressing and Siglec-8–expressing eosinophils,[37] confirming prior studies[38] regarding the influence of this cytokine on eosinophil-mediated inflammation.

As with eosinophils, mast cells are derived from pluripotent hematopoietic CD34[+] cells from the bone marrow,[39] but mast cells do not fully mature until they reach their final tissue destination, with the exception of mast cell leukemia. IL-3 and IL-6 increase early CD34[+] progenitor cell numbers and begin the differentiation process; however, it is binding of stem cell factor (SCF) to its receptor c-Kit (CD117) that is the master growth and differentiation factor for human mast cells (see **Fig. 1**).[40] SCF is produced primarily by stromal cells[41] and it can either be released as a soluble growth factor or expressed on the surface of these cells. It is the expression and binding of SCF at tissue sites that cause the CD34[+] precursor cells to arrest and terminally differentiate into mast cells.

## CYSTEINYL LEUKOTRIENE OVERPRODUCTION AND OVERRESPONSIVENESS IN ASPIRIN-EXACERBATED RESPIRATORY DISEASE

Arguably, the best-characterized molecules associated with AERD are the CysLTs. A unique characteristic of the disease is the overproduction of CysLTs in the resting state and a large surge in CysLT production in response to aspirin and other nonselective COX inhibitors that target COX-1.[42] Included in this list are the nonselective nonsteroidal antiinflammatory drugs (NSAIDs) as well as other inhibitors of COX-1.[43,44] The high CysLT levels in AERD reflect increased expression of the primary synthesis enzymes 5-lipoxygenase (5-LO) and, more importantly, leukotriene $C_4$ synthase (LTC$_4$S) (**Fig. 2**). Increased expression of these enzymes is observed in the lungs, sinuses, and nasal polyps of patients with AERD, with eosinophils and resident mast cells being the primary cells expressing the enzymes.[15,18,23,45]

Not only do patients with AERD produce more CysLTs but they also show an increased sensitivity to CysLTs.[46] Initially, 2 CysLT receptors were identified and were distinguished from each other by their differing potency for the CysLTs: CysLT1 receptors primarily respond to LTD$_4$, whereas CysLT2 receptors respond equally to LTD$_4$ and LTC$_4$. Neither receptor responds well to LTE$_4$. Acting through CysLT1 and inhibited by the CysLT2 receptor, CysLTs induce mast cell proliferation through activation of c-kit and extracellular signal-regulated kinase.[47] In AERD sinus tissue, high levels of CysLT1 were found compared with healthy tissue, and following aspirin desensitization the CysLT1 levels returned to normal.[48] CysLT1 receptors are also prominently expressed on airway smooth muscle[49] and these receptors mediate a portion of the CysLT-induced bronchospasm associated with aspirin challenges or desensitizations,[50–53] as shown by the ability of leukotriene receptor antagonists to attenuate much of the bronchospasm that occurs during these procedures.

Although these findings made it seem that CysLT1 was the only important leukotriene receptor in AERD, several observations suggested they were only partially

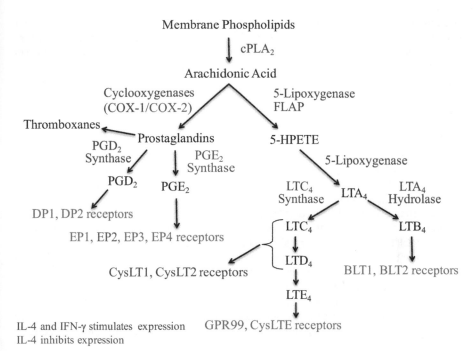

**Fig. 2.** Pathway depicting metabolites of arachidonic acid important in AERD. Following conversion to arachidonic acid by phospholipase A2, further processing occurs via either the prostaglandin pathway mediated by COX-1/COX-2 or the leukotriene pathway mediated by 5-LO. Red lettering shows genes inhibited by IL-4 and pink lettering shows genes stimulated by IL-4 and IFN-$\gamma$.

involved in the pathogenesis of disease. The most abundant leukotriene found in the circulation and airway is $LTE_4$, with $LTC_4$ and $LTD_4$ being rapidly converted to $LTE_4$, thus limiting their duration of action in vivo. Inhalation of $LTE_4$ by asthmatic patients and patients with AERD potentiates airway hyperresponsiveness to subsequent challenges with histamine, the effect of which could be blocked with indomethacin.[46,54,55] In the bronchial mucosa of asthmatics, inhalation of $LTE_4$, but not $LTD_4$, causes recruitment of eosinophils, basophils, and mast cells into the tissue.[56,57] Mice in which both the CysLT1 and CysLT2 receptors have been deleted show enhanced skin swelling in response to intracutaneous $LTE_4$ compared with mice with these genes intact.[58] These studies led to the exploration for and ultimate identification of additional CysLT receptors that selectively respond to $LTE_4$ (GPR99 and P2Y12).[58–61] The functional role of these $LTE_4$ receptors in AERD and the utility in targeting them as a therapeutic option are areas of active research, although diminished synthesis of CysLTs and, by extension, of $LTE_4$ could explain the superior efficacy of 5-lipoxygenase inhibitors in treating this disorder.[62]

## UNDERAPPRECIATED ROLE FOR PROSTAGLANDIN D₂ IN ASPIRIN-EXACERBATED RESPIRATORY DISEASE

$PGD_2$ and its metabolites have been found in blood and urine following aspirin challenge[10,12,63] and the conventional thought is that it is primarily mast cell derived; however, reports show that eosinophils are also a source.[64,65] Synthesis of $PGD_2$ is regulated by hematopoietic $PGD_2$ synthase (hPGDS) (see **Fig. 2**) and when secreted it binds 2 receptors, CRTH2 (DP2) and DP1, that are expressed on numerous cell types. Activities of $PGD_2$ binding include stimulation of cell migration (including eosinophils and innate lymphoid type 2 cells), bronchoconstriction, vasodilation (flushing), and cellular activation and differentiation.[66–69] A role for $PGD_2$ in the pathogenesis of AERD is supported by studies in chronic sinusitis. Expression of hPGDS has been observed in polyps, specifically in eosinophils.[65,70,71] The degree of hPGDS expression correlated with eosinophil number and severity of disease. These studies did not examine patients with AERD but, given the high levels of eosinophilic infiltrate in AERD tissue, it is likely that hPGDS levels would have correlated as well. Recent work from our laboratory showed that, among CRS syndromes, in AERD the highest levels of hPGDS transcripts and proteins expression were observed and that eosinophils were the predominant cell type in which expression was localized.[65] As discussed articles in this issue, aspirin desensitization followed by high-dose aspirin therapy is often used to treat AERD; however, not all patients tolerate the desensitization protocol. It has recently been shown that patients who cannot be desensitized express higher basal levels of $PGD_2$ (and thromboxane) in their serum and urine.[63] During the desensitization procedure, these patients had a surge of $PGD_2$ release but not thromboxane, whereas those who were successfully desensitized had decreased thromboxane and unchanged $PGD_2$ levels.[63] The correlation between $PGD_2$ and eosinophil number in the polyp tissue was not assessed. Baseline $PGD_2$ level may serve as a marker to identify patients who will successfully undergo desensitization.

## PROSTAGLANDIN $E_2$ AND PROSTAGLANDIN $E_2$ RECEPTOR DYSREGULATION IN ASPIRIN-EXACERBATED RESPIRATORY DISEASE

$PGE_2$ shows both proinflammatory and antiinflammatory functions, reflecting its ability to interact with 4 distinct receptors (EP1–EP4), each having various activating or inhibitory functions. However, it is the role of $PGE_2$ acting through antiinflammatory EP2 receptors to the block eosinophil and mast cell degranulation that is central to the pathogenesis of AERD. Patients with AERD constitutively produce low levels of $PGE_2$,[15,72] attenuating the antiinflammatory constraints provided by this lipid in this basal state. The further reduction of tissue $PGE_2$ concentrations by aspirin and other NSAIDs through COX-1 inhibition precipitates the activation of eosinophils and mast cells in AERD, as shown by the ability of inhaled $PGE_2$ to protect against these reactions.[73,74] This sensitivity of patients with AERD to low tissue $PGE_2$ concentrations is amplified by their reduced expression of the antiinflammatory EP2 receptor.[17] Serra-Pages and colleagues[75] showed that the ratio of EP2 to EP3 receptors on the surface of mast cells influences the activation potential of these cells when the high affinity immunoglobulin E receptor (FcεRI) is stimulated in a $PGE_2$-containing milieu. Through examination of various mast cell lines, the investigators found that patients with high levels of EP2 could suppress FcεRI activation in the presence of $PGE_2$, but when EP3 levels were high FcεRI activation of mast cells was enhanced. It is likely that the low EP2/EP3 ratio on mast cells and possibly eosinophils in AERD contributes to this disease because any $PGE_2$ that is available would preferentially signal through the EP3 receptor and activate these cells, thus contributing to the proinflammatory cascade.

Several studies have investigated the mechanism behind the reduced levels of $PGE_2$ in AERD and, perhaps not surprisingly, have correlated this with a decrease in the levels of the relevant upstream metabolic enzymes. The production of $PGE_2$ from arachidonic acid (see **Fig. 2**) involves the sequential synthesis of $PGG_2/PGH_2$ by the 2 COX enzymes (COX-1 and COX-2) followed by the synthesis of $PGE_2$ by the microsomal $PGE_2$ synthases (mPGES-1, mPGES-2) and cytosolic $PGE_2$ synthase (cPGES). It is mPGES-1 that is most relevant to $PGE_2$ production in inflammatory disorders such as AERD because it is the enzyme primarily functionally coupled to COX-2.[76] COX-2 messenger RNA (mRNA) and protein expression are markedly diminished in AERD.[15,16,77] Our studies have confirmed this diminished expression of COX-2.[78] We found no significant change in COX-1 and a trend toward diminished mPGES-1 expression and that this is driven in part by IL-4. Diminished COX-2 expression and the reduced capacity to synthesize $PGE_2$ contributes to the severity of inflammation observed in AERD and accentuates the sensitivity of these individuals to the further inhibition of $PGE_2$ synthesis associated with aspirin and other NSAIDs. With this shortage of COX-2, patients with AERD become dependent on COX-1 for the $PGE_2$ that is necessary to restrain mast cell and eosinophil activation. Thus, most patients with AERD tolerate selective COX-2 inhibitors,[79] supporting this concept regarding the unique importance of COX-1–derived $PGE_2$.

## CYTOKINE EXPRESSION IN ASPIRIN-EXACERBATED RESPIRATORY DISEASE

Numerous studies have examined the cytokine milieu found in the tissue of eosinophilic sinusitis and AERD. Many of these studies have reported expression of a Th2-like immune profile (IL-4, IL-13, and IL-5), similar to other allergic diseases with eosinophilic infiltrate, although few have specifically focused on AERD.[80–87] However, numerous observations suggest that, in contrast with patients with eosinophilic sinusitis who tolerate aspirin, AERD seems to have a mixed Th2-like and Th1-like cytokine milieu characterized by prominent expression of IFN-γ. The first study to suggest this examined patients with nonallergic sinusitis and showed enhanced IFN-γ expression in this cohort, a group in which AERD is likely to be overexpressed.[88] Since this initial report, high levels of IFN-γ in chronic sinusitis have been reported by other investigators, although patients with AERD were not specifically separated or recruited for the studies.[89] One study specifically addressed IFN-γ expression in AERD and found enhanced levels of IFN-γ in circulating CD8+ cells compared with aspirin-tolerant controls.[90] The concept that AERD reflects a mixed Th2-like and Th1-like cytokine profile was confirmed in our recent study in which NP tissue derived from patients with AERD was contrasted with tissue obtained from aspirin-tolerant and control subjects by the overexpression of IFN-γ mRNA transcripts and protein.[37] To our surprise, eosinophils themselves were the most important source for this cytokine, which is consistent with previous studies showing that IFN-γ can be expressed by eosinophils in substantial quantities.[91–93] In contrast with our findings, a recent report did not find increased levels of IFN-γ protein in nasal polyps from patients with AERD; however this group did not perform flow cytometry, immunohistochemistry, or quantitative polymerase chain reaction to verify their results.[87]

## CYTOKINE DYSREGULATION OF LEUKOTRIENE C4 SYNTHASE AND CYSTEINYL LEUKOTRIENE RECEPTORS

Under noninflammatory conditions, mast cells express moderate levels of $LTC_4S$ that can be increased greatly following stimulation by IL-4 (but not by IL-5 or IL-13).[94] It has also been observed that IFN-γ also has the capability of upregulating $LTC_4S$ expression in umbilical cord–derived mast cell progenitors (J Boyce, personal communication, 2013). Although mast cells are capable of synthesizing CysLTs, previous studies[23] have shown that eosinophils are the more important cell type overexpressing $LTC_4S$ in AERD. Examining a battery of cytokines (including IL-3, IL-4, IL-5, GM-CSF, IL-1, tumor necrosis factor alpha, and IFN-γ), the authors were unable to show an ability of any of these cytokines to modulate $LTC_4S$ expression on circulating eosinophils. This inability may be caused by their terminal differentiation state and short life span. The authors have also failed to show the ability of IL-4 to increase $LTC_4S$ expression on eosinophils differentiated from progenitors in the presence of IL-3 and IL-5. However, when the progenitors were incubated with IFN-γ during the differentiation stage, a significant increase in $LTC_4S$ expression was observed.[37] The increase in $LTC_4S$ expression translated into increased capacity of these newly differentiated eosinophils to secrete CysLTs on activation by aspirin.[13] Another mechanism of CysLT production involves the transcellular conversion of $LTA_4$ by adherent platelets expressing $LTC_4S$.[95] The frequencies of platelet-adherent eosinophils, neutrophils, and monocytes are markedly increased in the blood of patients with AERD. Any $LTA_4$ that is released into the extracellular space can be captured by the platelets and converted to CysLTs. It has been estimated that adherent platelets contribute up to 50% of the total $LTC_4S$ activity in blood and thus would represent a significant source of the CysLTs found in AERD.[95]

CysLT receptor expression is regulated by numerous cytokines, including IL-4 and IFN-γ but also IL-5 and IL-13. IL-4 increases expression of CysLT1 on mast cells[96,97] and monocytes.[98] In our studies, IL-4 also increased the expression of both CysLT1 and CysLT2 on T and B lymphocytes and eosinophils.[99] We also showed robust upregulation of CysLT1 and CysLT2 receptors in response to IFN-γ on T cells and eosinophils.[99] In recent studies, examination of eosinophils derived from CD34+ progenitors has also shown the ability of IFN-γ to upregulate CysLT1 and CysLT2 receptor expression.[37] There have been no reports of cytokine modulation of other CysLT receptors. In summary, in the AERD cytokine environment, both mast cells and eosinophils are primed to produce and respond to the CysLTs that are produced during the disease process.

## CYTOKINE DYSREGULATION OF PROSTAGLANDIN E2 SYNTHESIS AND EP2 RECEPTORS

Cytokine regulation of the $PGE_2$ synthesis pathway in AERD has not been thoroughly investigated. However, in other model systems, the influence of IL-4 on COX-2 expression has been reported. Inhibition of COX-2 expression by IL-4 was noted using peripheral blood monocytes, alveolar macrophages, and non–small cell lung cancer cells.[100–102] The authors performed studies on nasal polyp–derived fibroblasts and mononuclear phagocytic cells. Monocytes were used as representative inflammatory cells but also because $PGE_2$ is their dominant prostaglandin product. Similar to other findings, significant inhibition of COX-2 and also mPGES-1 (but not COX-1) mRNA and protein expression was observed following stimulation with IL-4 on both the monocytes and nasal polyp–derived fibroblasts.[78] Inhibition of COX-2 and mPGES-1 synergizes to result in dramatically less stimulated $PGE_2$ secretion by monocytes.[78] IL-13 has been reported to have a similar effect on airway epithelial cells.[103] Thus, in addition to enhancing the CysLT pathways, IL-4 and IL-13 contribute to the AERD phenotype through inhibition of the $PGE_2$ pathway. The role of IFN-γ modulation of the prostaglandin pathway is unclear because its action seems to be cell-type specific. IFN-γ can induce COX-2 mRNA in most inflammatory cells,[104,105] whereas it decreases COX-2 expression in placental[106] and intestinal epithelial cancer cells.[107] Actions of IFN-γ on other parts of the $PGE_2$ pathway have not been studied in detail.

## ACTIVATION OF EOSINOPHILS AND MAST CELLS BY ASPIRIN

It was unknown in AERD how aspirin triggered the release of proinflammatory mediators. Although, as noted, inhibition of COX releases the protective constraints provided by $PGE_2$, this alone does not explain the positive signaling driving cell activation. In a particularly robust murine model of AERD, aspirin sensitivity is induced by the knocking out of the mPGES-1 gene.[108] In this model, the positive (activating) signal is provided by allergic inflammation, a mechanism not likely to be relevant in AERD, at least in those patients with AERD who are not atopic. The authors speculated that aspirin and other NSAIDs had the inherent capacity to directly activate eosinophils and mast cells. When tested, both eosinophils and mast cells generated $Ca^{+2}$ fluxes following stimulation with water-soluble lysine aspirin (LysASA).[13] Similar results were observed with eosinophil activation measured by eosinophil derived neurotoxin (EDN) release and eosinophil and mast cell secretion of $PGD_2$.[13,65] When eosinophils from control, aspirin-tolerant patients, and patients with AERD were compared, no differences were observed in levels of mediator release. Our explanation as to why hypersensitivity reactions resulting from mediator release caused by aspirin/NSAIDs are not observed in these control cohorts reflects alterations in their $PGE_2$ sensitivity, specifically the decreased capacity to produce and respond to this antiinflammatory mediator observed in AERD. We speculate that the higher expression of $PGE_2$, as well as its antiinflammatory EP2 receptor, acts to prevent the acute reactions to aspirin/NSAIDs in controls and aspirin-tolerant asthmatics.[20,73] An additional explanation for the absence of clinical symptoms in these control cohorts is that, when activated with aspirin, their circulating eosinophils produced very low levels of CysLTs,[13] in contrast with the robust levels found in patients with AERD following aspirin ingestion.[42] As mentioned earlier, AERD sinonasal and lung tissue is characterized by high numbers of eosinophilic hematopoietic progenitor ($CD34^+IL-5R\alpha^+$) cells.[28,109] We therefore investigated whether eosinophils differentiated from progenitor cells in the presence of IFN-$\gamma$ would recapitulate the sensitivity to aspirin shown by tissue eosinophils in vivo in AERD. After maturation with IFN-$\gamma$, the mature eosinophils showed increased gene expression for both $LTC_4S$ and hPGDS.[13,65] Consistent with the increase in $LTC_4S$ gene expression, CysLT secretion was dramatically increased on LysASA activation.[13] In addition to increased CysLT production, these IFN-$\gamma$ matured eosinophils showed enhanced $PGD_2$ production when stimulated with LysASA.[65]

## SUMMARY: TOWARD A GENERALIZED MODEL FOR THE INDUCTION OF THE ASPIRIN-EXACERBATED RESPIRATORY DISEASE PHENOTYPE

Although it has been understood for many years that aspirin causes reactions and that AERD is a debilitating disease, the exact mechanisms driving AERD and how to treat it are still largely unknown. Our work and that of others have shown the importance of both eosinophils and mast cells as drivers of the disease leading to increased expression of proinflammatory mediators and reflecting the loss of protective $PGE_2$. The ultimate result is constitutive overproduction of and overresponsiveness to mediators by eosinophils and mast cells in the basal state in AERD, with the uncontrolled release of mediators when these cells are directly triggered by aspirin. The increased recognition of the cellular components and mechanisms of action in AERD provides an opportunity to develop alternative targeted therapeutic approaches designed to dampen the severe impacts of this disease.

## REFERENCES

1. Samter M, Beers RF Jr. Intolerance to aspirin. Clinical studies and consideration of its pathogenesis. Ann Intern Med 1968;68:975–83.

2. Mattos JL, Woodard CR, Payne SC. Trends in common rhinologic illnesses: analysis of U.S. healthcare surveys 1995-2007. Int Forum Allergy Rhinol 2011; 1:3–12.

3. Rajan JP, Wineinger NE, Stevenson DD, et al. Prevalence of aspirin-exacerbated respiratory disease among asthmatic patients: a meta-analysis of the literature. J Allergy Clin Immunol 2015;135:676–81.e1.

4. Szczeklik A, Stevenson DD. Aspirin-induced asthma: advances in pathogenesis and management. J Allergy Clin Immunol 1999;104:5–13.

5. Szczeklik A, Nizankowska E. Clinical features and diagnosis of aspirin induced asthma. Thorax 2000;55:S42–4.

6. Berges-Gimeno MP, Simon RA, Stevenson DD. The natural history and clinical characteristics of aspirin-exacerbated respiratory disease. Ann Allergy Asthma Immunol 2002;89:474–8.

7. Vally H, Taylor ML, Thompson PJ. The prevalence of aspirin intolerant asthma (AIA) in Australian asthmatic patients. Thorax 2002;57:569–74.

8. Mascia K, Borish L, Patrie J, et al. Chronic hyperplastic eosinophilic sinusitis as a predictor of aspirin-exacerbated respiratory disease. Ann Allergy Asthma Immunol 2005;94:652–7.

9. Mascia K, Haselkorn T, Deniz YM, et al. Aspirin sensitivity and severity of asthma: evidence for irreversible airway obstruction in patients with severe or difficult-to-treat asthma. J Allergy Clin Immunol 2005;116:970–5.

10. Fischer AR, Rosenberg MA, Lilly CM, et al. Direct evidence for a role of the mast cell in the nasal response to aspirin in aspirin-sensitive asthma. J Allergy Clin Immunol 1994;94:1046–56.

11. Daffern PJ, Muilenburg D, Hugli TE, et al. Association of urinary leukotriene E4 excretion during aspirin challenges with severity of respiratory responses. J Allergy Clin Immunol 1999;104:559–64.

12. Bochenek G, Nagraba K, Nizankowska E, et al. A controlled study of 9alpha,11-beta-PGF2 (a prostaglandin D2 metabolite) in plasma and urine of patients with bronchial asthma and healthy controls after aspirin challenge. J Allergy Clin Immunol 2003;111:743–9.

13. Steinke JW, Negri J, Liu L, et al. Aspirin activation of eosinophils and mast cells: implications in the pathogenesis of aspirin-exacerbated respiratory disease. J Immunol 2014;193:41–7.

14. Antczak A, Montuschi P, Kharitonov S, et al. Increased exhaled cysteinyl-leukotrienes and 8-isoprostane in aspirin-induced asthma. Am J Respir Crit Care Med 2002;166:301–6.

15. Perez-Novo CA, Watelet JB, Claeys C, et al. Prostaglandin, leukotriene, and lipoxin balance in chronic rhinosinusitis with and without nasal polyposis. J Allergy Clin Immunol 2005;115:1189–96.

16. Picado C, Fernandez-Morata JC, Juan M, et al. Cyclooxygenase-2 mRNA is downexpressed in nasal polyps from aspirin-sensitive asthmatics. Am J Respir Crit Care Med 1999;160:291–6.

17. Ying S, Meng Q, Scadding G, et al. Aspirin-sensitive rhinosinusitis is associated with reduced E-prostanoid 2 receptor expression on nasal mucosal inflammatory cells. J Allergy Clin Immunol 2006;117:312–8.

18. Steinke JW, Bradley D, Arango P, et al. Cysteinyl leukotriene expression in chronic hyperplastic sinusitis-nasal polyposis: importance to eosinophilia and asthma. J Allergy Clin Immunol 2003;111:342–9.

19. Beller TC, Friend DS, Maekawa A, et al. Cysteinyl leukotriene 1 receptor controls the severity of chronic pulmonary inflammation and fibrosis. Proc Natl Acad Sci U S A 2004;101:3047–52.

20. Steinke JW. Editorial: Yin-Yang of EP receptor expression. J Leukoc Biol 2012; 92:1129–31.

21. Adamjee J, Suh YJ, Park HS, et al. Expression of 5-lipoxygenase and cyclooxygenase pathway enzymes in nasal polyps of patients with aspirin-intolerant asthma. J Pathol 2006;209:392–9.

22. Payne SC, Early SB, Huyett P, et al. Evidence for distinct histologic profile of nasal polyps with and without eosinophilia. Laryngoscope 2011;121:2262–7.

23. Cowburn AS, Sladek K, Soja J, et al. Overexpression of leukotriene C4 synthase in bronchial biopsies from patients with aspirin-intolerant asthma. J Clin Invest 1998;101:834–46.

24. Park HS, Nahm DH, Park K, et al. Immunohistochemical characterization of cellular infiltrate in nasal polyp from aspirin-sensitive asthmatic patients. Ann Allergy Asthma Immunol 1998;81:219–24.

25. Corrigan CJ, Napoli RL, Meng Q, et al. Reduced expression of the prostaglandin E2 receptor E-prostanoid 2 on bronchial mucosal leukocytes in patients with aspirin-sensitive asthma. J Allergy Clin Immunol 2012;129:1636–46.

26. Boyce JA, Friend D, Matsumoto R, et al. Differentiation in vitro of hybrid eosinophil/basophile granulocytes: autocrine function of an eosinophil intermediate. J Exp Med 1995;182:49–57.

27. Denburg JA, Sehmi R, Saito H, et al. Systemic aspects of allergic disease: bone marrow responses. J Allergy Clin Immunol 2000;106:S242–6.

28. Kim YK, Uno M, Hamilos DL, et al. Immunolocalization of CD34 in nasal polyp. Effect of topical corticosteroids. Am J Respir Cell Mol Biol 1999;20:388–97.

29. Nerlov C, Graf T. PU.1 induces myeloid lineage commitment in multipotent hematopoietic progenitors. Genes Dev 1998;12:2403–12.

30. Nerlov C, McNagny KM, Doderlein G, et al. Distinct C/EBP functions are required for eosinophil lineage commitment and maturation. Genes Dev 1998; 12:2413–23.

31. McNagny K, Graf T. Making eosinophils through subtle shifts in transcription factor expression. J Exp Med 2002;195:F43–7.

32. Hirasawa R, Shimizu R, Takahashi S, et al. Essential and instructive roles of GATA factors in eosinophil development. J Exp Med 2002;195:1379–86.

33. Nishijima I, Nakahata T, Hirabayashi Y, et al. A human-GM-CSF receptor expressed in transgenic mice stimulates proliferation and differentiation of hemopoietic progenitors to all lineages in response to human GM-CSF. Mol Cell Biol 1995;6:497–508.

34. Sanderson CJ. Interleukin-5, eosinophils, and disease. Blood 1992;79:3101–9.

35. Collins PD, Marleau S, Griffiths-Johnson DA, et al. Cooperation between interleukin-5 and the chemokine eotaxin to induce eosinophil accumulation in vivo. J Exp Med 1995;182:1169–74.

36. Milanovic M, Terszowski G, Struck D, et al. IFN consensus sequence binding protein (ICSBP) is critical for eosinophil development. J Immunol 2008;181: 5045–53.

37. Steinke JW, Liu L, Huyett P, et al. Prominent role of interferon-γ in aspirin-exacerbated respiratory disease. J Allergy Clin Immunol 2013;132:856–65.e3.

38. de Bruin AM, Buitenhuis M, van der Sluijs KF, et al. Eosinophil differentiation in the bone marrow is inhibited by T cell-derived IFN-gamma. Blood 2010;116: 2559–69.

39. Kirshenbaum AS, Goff JP, Semere T, et al. Demonstration that human mast cells arise from a progenitor cell population that is CD34(+), c-kit(+), and expresses aminopeptidase N (CD13). Blood 1999;94:2333–42.

40. Kirshenbaum AS, Goff JP, Kessler SW, et al. Effect of IL-3 and stem cell factor on the appearance of human basophils and mast cells from CD34+ pluripotent progenitor cells. J Immunol 1992;148:772–7.

41. Anderson DM, Lyman SD, Baird A, et al. Molecular cloning of mast cell growth factor, a hematopoietin that is active in both membrane bound and soluble forms. Cell 1990;63:235–43.

42. Christie PE, Tagari P, Ford-Hutchinson AW, et al. Urinary leukotriene E4 concentrations increase after aspirin challenge in aspirin-sensitive asthmatic subjects. Am Rev Respir Dis 1991;143:1025–9.

43. Cardet JC, White AA, Barrett NA, et al. Alcohol-induced respiratory symptoms are common in patients with aspirin exacerbated respiratory disease. J Allergy Clin Immunol Pract 2014;2:208–13.

44. Payne SC. Alcohol-induced respiratory symptoms are common in patients with aspirin exacerbated respiratory disease. J Allergy Clin Immunol Pract 2014;2:644.

45. Sampson AP, Cowburn AS, Sladek K. Profound overexpression of leukotriene C4 synthase in bronchial biopsies from aspirin-intolerant asthmatic patients. Int Arch Allergy Immunol 1997;113:355–7.

46. Arm JP, O'Hickey S, Spur BW, et al. Airway responsiveness to histamine and leukotriene E4 in subjects with aspirin-induced asthma. Am Rev Respir Dis 1989;140:148–53.

47. Jiang Y, Borrelli LA, Kanaoka Y, et al. CysLT2 receptors interact with CysLT1 receptors and down-modulate cysteinyl leukotriene dependent mitogenic responses of mast cells. Blood 2007;110:3263–70.

48. Sousa AR, Parikh A, Scadding G, et al. Leukotriene-receptor expression on nasal mucosal inflammatory cells in aspirin-sensitive rhinosinusitis. N Engl J Med 2002;347:1493–9.

49. Lynch KR, O'Neill GP, Liu Q, et al. Characterization of the human cysteinyl leukotriene CysLT1 receptor. Nature 1999;399:789–93.

50. Christie PE, Smith CM, Lee TH. The potent and selective sulfidopeptide leukotriene antagonists, SK&F 104353, inhibits aspirin-induced asthma. Am Rev Respir Dis 1991;144:957–8.

51. Dahlen B. Treatment of aspirin-intolerant asthma with antileukotrienes. Am J Respir Crit Care Med 2000;161:S137–41.

52. Walch L, Norel X, Back M, et al. Pharmacological evidence for a novel cysteinyl-leukotriene receptor subtype in human pulmonary artery smooth muscle. Br J Pharmacol 2002;137:1339–45.

53. White A, Bigby T, Stevenson D. Intranasal ketorolac challenge for the diagnosis of aspirin-exacerbated respiratory disease. Ann Allergy Asthma Immunol 2006; 97:190–5.

54. Christie PE, Hawksworth R, Spur BW, et al. Effect of indomethacin on leukotriene4-induced histamine hyperresponsiveness in asthmatic subjects. Am Rev Respir Dis 1992;146:1506–10.

55. Christie PE, Schmitz-Schumann M, Spur BW, et al. Airway responsiveness to leukotriene C4 (LTC4), leukotriene E4 (LTE4) and histamine in aspirin-sensitive asthmatic subjects. Eur Respir J 1993;6:1468–73.

56. Laitinen LA, Laitinen A, Haahtela T, et al. Leukotriene E4 and granulocytic infiltration into asthmatic airways. Lancet 1993;341:989–90.

57. Gauvreau GM, Parameswaran KN, Watson RM, et al. Inhaled leukotriene E(4), but not leukotriene D(4), increased airway inflammatory cells in subjects with atopic asthma. Am J Respir Crit Care Med 2001;164:1495–500.
58. Maekawa A, Kanaoka Y, Xing W, et al. Functional recognition of a distinct receptor preferential for leukotriene E4 in mice lacking the cysteinyl leukotriene 1 and 2 receptors. Proc Natl Acad Sci U S A 2008;105:16695–700.
59. Nonaka Y, Hiramoto T, Fujita N. Identification of endogenous surrogate ligands for human P2Y12 receptors by in silico and in vitro methods. Biochem Biophys Res Commun 2005;337:281–8.
60. Paruchuri S, Tashimo H, Feng C, et al. Leukotriene E4-induced pulmonary inflammation is mediated by the P2Y12 receptor. J Exp Med 2009;206:2543–55.
61. Kanaoka Y, Maekawa A, Austen KF. Identification of GPR99 protein as a potential third cysteinyl leukotriene receptor with a preference for leukotriene E4 ligand. J Biol Chem 2013;288:10967–72.
62. Dahlen B, Nizankowska E, Szczeklik A. Benefits from adding the 5-lipoxygenase inhibitor zileuton to conventional therapy in aspirin-intolerant asthmatics. Am J Respir Crit Care Med 1998;157:1187–94.
63. Cahill KN, Bensko JC, Boyce JA, et al. Prostaglandin D(2): a dominant mediator of aspirin-exacerbated respiratory disease. J Allergy Clin Immunol 2015;135:245–52.
64. Luna-Gomes T, Magalhaes KG, Mesquita-Santos FP, et al. Eosinophils as a novel cell source of prostaglandin D2: autocrine role in allergic inflammation. J Immunol 2011;187:6518–26.
65. Feng X, Negri J, Baker MG, et al. Eosinophil production of PGD2 in aspirin-exacerbated respiratory disease. J Allergy Clin Immunol 2016. in press.
66. Hirai H, Tanaka K, Yoshie O, et al. Prostaglandin D2 selectively induces chemotaxis in T helper type 2 cells, eosinophils, and basophils via seventransmembrane receptor CRTH2. J Exp Med 2001;193:255–61.
67. Satoh T, Moroi R, Aritake K, et al. Prostaglandin D2 plays an essential role in chronic allergic inflammation of the skin via CRTH2 receptor. J Immunol 2006;177:2621–9.
68. Schratl P, Royer JF, Kostenis E, et al. The role of the prostaglandin D2 receptor, DP, in eosinophil trafficking. J Immunol 2007;179:4792–9.
69. Stinson SE, Amrani Y, Brightling CE. D prostanoid receptor 2 (chemoattractant receptor-homologous molecule expressed on TH2 cells) protein expression in asthmatic patients and its effects on bronchial epithelial cells. J Allergy Clin Immunol 2015;135:395–406.
70. Okano M, Fujiwara T, Yamamoto M, et al. Role of prostaglandin D2 and E2 terminal synthases in chronic rhinosinusitis. Clin Exp Allergy 2006;36:1028–38.
71. Hyo S, Kawata R, Kadoyama K, et al. Expression of prostaglandin D2 synthase in activated eosinophils in nasal polyps. Arch Otolaryngol Head Neck Surg 2007;133:693–700.
72. Schmid M, Gode U, Schafer D, et al. Arachidonic acid metabolism in nasal tissue and peripheral blood cells in aspirin intolerant asthmatics. Acta Otolaryngol 1999;119:277–80.
73. Sestini P, Armetti L, Gambaro G, et al. Inhaled PgE2 prevents aspirin-induced bronchoconstriction and urinary LTE4 excretion in aspirin-sensitive asthma. Am J Respir Crit Care Med 1996;153:572–5.
74. Feng C, Beller EM, Bagga S, et al. Human mast cells express multiple EP receptors for prostaglandin E2 that differentially modulate activation responses. Blood 2006;107:3243–50.

75. Serra-Pages M, Olivera A, Torres R, et al. E-prostanoid 2 receptors dampen mast cell degranulation via cAMP/PKA-mediated suppression of IgE-dependent signaling. J Leukoc Biol 2012;92(6):1155–65.
76. Murakami M, Nakashima K, Kamei D, et al. Cellular prostaglandin E2 production by membrane-bound prostaglandin E synthase-2 via both cyclooxygenases-1 and -2. J Biol Chem 2003;278:37937–47.
77. Gosepath J, Brieger J, Mann WJ. New immunohistologic findings on the differential role of cyclooxygenase 1 and cyclooxygenase 2 in nasal polyposis. Am J Rhinol 2005;19:111–6.
78. Steinke JW, Culp JA, Kropf E, et al. Modulation by aspirin of nuclear phospho-signal transducer and activator of transcription 6 expression: possible role in therapeutic benefit associated with aspirin desensitization. J Allergy Clin Immunol 2009;124:724–30.e4.
79. Stevenson DD, Szczeklik A. Clinical and pathologic perspectives on aspirin sensitivity and asthma. J Allergy Clin Immunol 2006;118:773–86 [quiz: 87–8].
80. Bachert C, Wagenmann M, Hauser U, et al. IL-5 synthesis is upregulated in human nasal polyp tissue. J Allergy Clin Immunol 1997;99:837–42.
81. Bachert C, Gevaert P, van Cauwenberge P. Nasal polyposis - A new concept on the formation of polyps. Allergy Clin Immunol Int 1999;11:130–5.
82. Minshall EM, Cameron L, Lavigne F, et al. Eotaxin mRNA and protein expression in chronic sinusitis and allergen-induced nasal responses in seasonal allergic rhinitis. Am J Respir Cell Mol Biol 1997;17:683–90.
83. Hamilos DL, Leung DYM, Huston DP, et al. IL-5, and RANTES immunoreactivity and mRNA expression in chronic hyperplastic sinusitis with nasal polyposis. Clin Exp Allergy 1998;28:1145–52.
84. Kamil A, Ghaffar O, Lavigne F, et al. Comparison of inflammatory cell profile and Th2 cytokine expression in the ethmoid sinuses, maxillary sinuses, and turbinates of atopic subjects with chronic sinusitis. Otolaryngol Head Neck Surg 1998;18:804–9.
85. Riechelmann H, Deutschle T, Rozsasi A, et al. Nasal biomarker profiles in acute and chronic rhinosinusitis. Clin Exp Allergy 2005;35:1186–91.
86. Van Bruaene N, Perez-Novo CA, Basinski TM, et al. T-cell regulation in chronic paranasal sinus disease. J Allergy Clin Immunol 2008;121:1435–41, 41.e1–3.
87. Stevens WW, Ocampo CJ, Berdnikovs S, et al. Cytokines in chronic rhinosinusitis. role in eosinophilia and aspirin-exacerbated respiratory disease. Am J Respir Crit Care Med 2015;192:682–94.
88. Hamilos DL, Leung DYM, Wood R, et al. Evidence for distinct cytokine expression in allergic versus nonallergic chronic sinusitis. J Allergy Clin Immunol 1995;96:537–44.
89. Van Zele T, Claeys S, Gevaert P, et al. Differentiation of chronic sinus diseases by measurement of inflammatory mediators. Allergy 2006;61:1280–9.
90. Shome GP, Tarbox J, Shearer M, et al. Cytokine expression in peripheral blood lymphocytes before and after aspirin desensitization in aspirin-exacerbated respiratory disease. Allergy Asthma Proc 2007;28:706–10.
91. Kanda A, Driss V, Hornez N, et al. Eosinophil-derived IFN-γ induces airway hyperresponsiveness and lung inflammation in the absence of lymphocytes. J Allergy Clin Immunol 2009;124:573–82.
92. Akuthota P, Xenakis JJ, Weller PF. Eosinophils: offenders or general bystanders in allergic airway disease and pulmonary immunity? J Innate Immun 2011;3:113–9.

93. Spencer LA, Szela CT, Perez SAC, et al. Human eosinophils constitutively express multiple Th1, Th2, and immunoregulatory cytokines that are secreted rapidly and differentially. J Leukoc Biol 2009;85:117–23.

94. Hsieh FH, Lam BK, Penrose JF, et al. T helper cell type 2 cytokines coordinately regulate immunoglobulin E-dependent cysteinyl leukotriene production by human cord blood-derived mast cells: profound induction of leukotriene C4 synthase expression by interleukin 4. J Exp Med 2001;193:123–33.

95. Laidlaw TM, Kidder MS, Bhattacharyya N, et al. Cysteinyl leukotriene overproduction in aspirin-exacerbated respiratory disease is driven by platelet-adherent leukocytes. Blood 2012;119:3790–8.

96. Mellor EA, Austen KF, Boyce JA. Cysteinyl leukotrienes and uridine diphosphate induce cytokine generation by human mast cells through an interleukin 4-regulated pathway that is inhibited by leukotriene receptor antagonists. J Exp Med 2002;195:583–92.

97. Mellor EA, Frank N, Soler D, et al. Expression of the type 2 receptor for cysteinyl leukotrienes (CysLT2R) by human mast cells: Functional distinction from CysLT1R. Proc Natl Acad Sci U S A 2003;100:11589–93.

98. Thivierge M, Stankova J, Rola-Pleszczynski M. IL-13 and IL-4 up-regulate cysteinyl leukotriene 1 receptor expression in human monocytes and macrophages. J Immunol 2001;167:2855–60.

99. Early SB, Barekzi E, Negri J, et al. Concordant modulation of cysteinyl leukotriene receptor expression by IL-4 and IFN-g on peripheral immune cells. Am J Respir Cell Mol Biol 2007;36:715–20.

100. Yano T, Hopkins HA, Hempel SL, et al. Interleukin-4 inhibits lipopolysaccharide-induced expression of prostaglandin H synthase-2 in human alveolar macrophages. J Cell Physiol 1995;165:77–82.

101. Dworski R, Sheller JR. Differential sensitivities of human blood monocytes and alveolar macrophages to the inhibition of prostaglandin endoperoxide synthase-2 by interleukin-4. Prostaglandins 1997;53:237–51.

102. Cui X, Yang SC, Sharma S, et al. IL-4 regulates COX-2 and PGE2 production in human non-small cell lung cancer. Biochem Biophys Res Commun 2006;343:995–1001.

103. Trudeau J, Hu H, Chibana K, et al. Selective downregulation of prostaglandin $E_2$-related pathways by the $T_H2$ cytokine IL-13. J Allergy Clin Immunol 2006;117:1446–54.

104. Matsuura H, Sakaue M, Subbaramaiah K, et al. Regulation of cyclooxygenase-2 by interferon gamma and transforming growth factor alpha in normal human epidermal keratinocytes and squamous carcinoma cells. Role of mitogen-activated protein kinases. J Biol Chem 1999;274:29138–48.

105. Kim J, Yoon Y, Jeoung D, et al. Interferon-gamma stimulates human follicular dendritic cell-like cells to produce prostaglandins via the JAK-STAT pathway. Mol Immunol 2015;66:189–96.

106. Hanna N, Bonifacio L, Reddy P, et al. IFN-gamma-mediated inhibition of COX-2 expression in the placenta from term and preterm labor pregnancies. Am J Reprod Immunol 2004;51:311–8.

107. Klampfer L, Huang J, Kaler P, et al. STAT1-independent inhibition of cyclooxygenase-2 expression by IFNgamma; a common pathway of IFNgamma-mediated gene repression but not gene activation. Oncogene 2007;26:2071–81.

108. Liu T, Laidlaw TM, Katz HR, et al. Prostaglandin E2 deficiency causes a phenotype of aspirin sensitivity that depends on platelets and cysteinyl leukotrienes. Proc Natl Acad Sci U S A 2013;110:16987–92.

109. Denburg JA. Haemopoietic mechanisms in nasal polyposis and asthma. Thorax 2000;55:S24–5.

# Mechanisms of Benefit with Aspirin Therapy in Aspirin-Exacerbated Respiratory Disease

Jennifer Hill, MD[a], Trever Burnett, MD[b], Rohit Katial, MD[c],*

## KEYWORDS

- Aspirin-exacerbated respiratory disease (AERD) • Aspirin desensitization
- Mechanisms of action • Cysteinyl leukotrienes (CysLTs) • Cytokines
- Interleukin 4 (IL-4) • Signal transducer and activator of transcription 6 (STAT6)
- Prostaglandin D2

## KEY POINTS

- Aspirin-exacerbated respiratory disease (AERD) is characterized by severe, persistent asthma, hyperplastic eosinophilic sinusitis with nasal polyps, and intolerance to aspirin and other nonsteroidal anti-inflammatory drugs.
- Aspirin desensitization is an effective therapeutic option in carefully selected patients; however, the mechanisms behind the effects of aspirin desensitization remain poorly understood.
- AERD is associated with an overexpression of cysteinyl leukotrienes (CysLTs), with marked upregulation of CysLT receptors.
- Despite increased knowledge about the pathophysiology underlying AERD, the mechanisms behind the therapeutic effects of aspirin desensitization remain poorly understood.
- Recent studies suggest that the clinical benefits of aspirin desensitization may occur through direct inhibition of tyrosine kinases and the signal transducer and activator of transcription 6 pathway, with resultant inhibition of interleukin 4 production.
- A reduction in prostaglandin D2, as a consequence of aspirin desensitization, may also produce clinical benefit in AERD by precluding recruitment of PGD2 responsive effector cells to the airways.

Funding Sources: None.
Conflict of Interest: None.
[a] Adult Program, Division of Allergy and Immunology, National Jewish Health, University of Colorado, 1400 Jackson Street, K624, Denver, CO 80206, USA; [b] Northwest Asthma and Allergy Center, 9725 3rd Avenue Northeast, Suite 500, Northgate Executive Center II, Seattle, WA 98115, USA; [c] Division of Allergy and Immunology, National Jewish Health, University of Colorado, 1400 Jackson Street, K624, Denver, CO 80206, USA
* Corresponding author.
E-mail address: KatialR@NJHealth.org

Immunol Allergy Clin N Am 36 (2016) 735–747
http://dx.doi.org/10.1016/j.iac.2016.06.011
0889-8561/16/© 2016 Elsevier Inc. All rights reserved.
immunology.theclinics.com

## INTRODUCTION

Aspirin was first synthesized by Felix Hoffman in 1897 and was marketed by Bayer as an anti-inflammatory drug in 1899.[1] Idiosyncratic reactions to aspirin were reported shortly after the drug's development, although Widal and colleagues[2] was the first to describe aspirin challenges and desensitization for patients with the syndrome of asthma, nasal polyposis, and aspirin intolerance in 1922. Later, following works by Samter and Beers,[3] the condition was termed Samter triad because of the association of these 3 overlapping conditions, although aspirin-exacerbated respiratory disease (AERD) is now the preferred nomenclature. Stevenson and colleagues[4] reported the successful treatment of AERD with aspirin desensitization followed by daily aspirin therapy. Their study demonstrated significant clinical improvement in nasal symptoms and requirement for nasal steroids following aspirin desensitization.[5] Symptom improvement in AERD has been reported to occur as early as 4 weeks after initiation of aspirin therapy, and long-term benefits include considerable reductions in the number of sinus infections and surgeries, hospitalizations for asthma, and use of systemic steroids.[6,7] Despite these data, which support the clinical benefit, the mechanisms of aspirin therapy remain the least understood aspect of the disease.

Central to AERD is the dysregulation of endogenous inflammatory and anti-inflammatory mediators produced from the metabolism of arachidonic acid (also known as eicosatetraenoic acid).[8] Abnormalities in these eicosanoid mediators (including leukotrienes [LTs], prostaglandins [PGs], lipoxins [LXs], and their respective receptors) have all been implicated in the pathogenesis of AERD.[9] Evidence reveals that baseline expression of CysLTs is increased in patients with AERD and these levels further increase in response to cyclooxygenase-1 (COX-1) inhibitor challenge.[10-16] Concomitantly, in tissue mast cells (MC) and eosinophils, there is an increased expression of $LTC_4$ synthase ($LTC_4 S$), the rate limiting enzyme in CysLT synthesis.[17,18] $CysLT_1$ receptor expression is likewise elevated at baseline.[19] Reduction in the synthesis and under expression of $PGE_2$, an important inhibitor of 5-LO and thus leukotriene production, also contributes to AERD pathogenesis.[20]

Recent studies suggest that the AERD phenotype may result from a contribution of the cytokine interleukin 4 (IL-4), particularly in the presence of IFN-$\gamma$.[21-24] Aspirin desensitization and continued therapy leads to an immediate improvement in the dysregulation of arachidonic acid metabolism. During desensitization, urine $LTE_4$ ($uLTE_4$) levels initially increase following aspirin ingestion but subsequently decrease to basal levels with continued treatment.[25] $CysLT_1$ receptor expression is also decreased following desensitization.[19] Concomitantly, there is reduction of IL-4 induced expression of leukotrienes, which may occur through direct inhibition of the IL-4–activated signal transducer and activator of transcription 6 (STAT6) pathway.[21,24,26,27] A reduction in prostaglandin $D_2$, as a consequence of aspirin desensitization, may also produce clinical benefit in AERD by precluding recruitment of $PGD_2$ responsive effector cells to the airways.[28,29] These findings give insight into the mechanism of aspirin desensitization and are the subject of this review.

## DESENSITIZATION EFFECTS ON PRODUCTS OF ARACHIDONIC ACID METABOLISM

$LTE_4$ is the most stable of the CysLTs and mediates many of the principal aspects of AERD, including bronchial constriction, hyperresponsiveness, eosinophilia, and increased vascular permeability.[30] Nasser and colleagues[25] studied the effects of aspirin desensitization on $uLTE_4$ concentrations in 9 patients with AERD. $uLTE_4$ levels were measured before and then at specific time intervals for 9 hours after aspirin administration. Comparison was made between the following:

1. An initial dose of aspirin (mean of approximately 90 mg), which resulted in a 15% reduction in $FEV_1$ (forced expiratory volume in first second of expiration);
2. 600-mg aspirin 24 hours after desensitization; and
3. The 600-mg maintenance dose at least 2 months after desensitization.

Before desensitization, the initial dose of aspirin resulted in a sevenfold increase in $uLTE_4$ from baseline levels at 3 hours after ingestion. The comparable increases were threefold after initial desensitization and twofold with maintenance aspirin dosing (**Fig. 1**). Overall, the aspirin provoked increase in $uLTE_4$ production was reduced by 82% and 86% after initial desensitization and with continued maintenance therapy, respectively. The maximum reduction in $FEV_1$ was also improved from 15.3% ± 3.9% after initial aspirin dosing, to 3.3% ± 2.4% after initial desensitization and 7.4% ± 4.5% with continued therapy (**Fig. 2**). Additional studies also showed that continued aspirin therapy after successful desensitization results in a 20-fold reduction in bronchial responsiveness to inhaled $LTE_4$.[31,32] Together these findings demonstrate that in patients with AERD, aspirin desensitization results in both decreased production of $LTE_4$ and reduced airway responsiveness to $LTE_4$.

$LTB_4$, which is metabolized from $LTA_4$ via $LTA_4$ hydrolase, is a potent chemotactic factor for eosinophils and neutrophils and contributes to the chronic inflammation seen in AERD.[8] Juergens and colleagues[33] studied the release of $LTB_4$ and $LTC_4$ from calcium ionophore-stimulated peripheral blood monocytes from patients with AERD and normal volunteers before and after desensitization. Consistent with previous studies, patients with AERD had increased baseline levels of $TXB_2$, $LTB_4$, and $LTC_4$. After aspirin desensitization, $TXB_2$ was almost completely suppressed in both groups. $LTB_4$ release was reduced by 42% in the AERD group. Clinically, 8 of the 10 patients with AERD were taking prednisone before aspirin challenge. After desensitization, prednisone dosing was reduced, with an 85% reduction in average steroid dose (10.4 ± 2.2 mg/d to 1.6 ± 2.8 mg/d).

One of the major COX products of mast cells, $PGD_2$, as well as its metabolite, 9 alpha,11 Beta-$PGF_2$, is higher at baseline in patients with AERD than in aspirin-tolerant

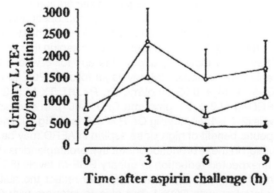

**Fig. 1.** $uLTE_4$ levels in 5 patients for 9 hours after challenge at the threshold dose of aspirin (○) and with 600 mg aspirin at 24 hours (△) and at 9 (3.2) months after aspirin desensitization (●). Each point is mean ± SEM. (*From* Nasser S, Patel M, Bell G, et al. The effect of aspirin desensitization on urinary leukotriene E4 concentrations in aspirin-sensitive asthma. Am J Respir Crit Care Med 1995;151:1329; with permission.)

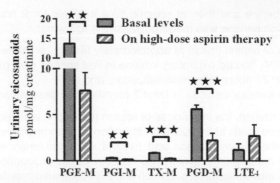

**Fig. 2.** Effect of high-dose aspirin therapy on urinary eicosanoid levels in patients with AERD. Urinary eicosanoid levels of patients with AERD are shown at baseline before aspirin and after 650 mg of twice-daily aspirin therapy for 8 weeks. Data are expressed as means ± SEMs. **$P<.01$ and ***$P<.001$. (*From* Cahill KN, Bensko JC, Boyce JA, et al. Prostaglandin D2: a dominant mediator of aspirin-exacerbated respiratory disease. J Allergy Clin Immunol 2015;135(1):245–52; with permission.)

asthmatic patients and healthy control subjects. Interestingly, these levels increase further in patients with AERD following ASA challenge, indicating mast cell activation.[28,29,34] $PGD_2$ is a potent chemotactic for $T_H2$ cells, innate helper lymphoid cells, basophils, and eosinophils, all of which express the D prostanoid 2/chemokine receptor homologous molecule (DP2/CRTH2) receptor.[35] $PGD_2$, through DP2/CRTH2, may promote the persistent eosinophilic inflammation of the respiratory tract that characterizes AERD.[28,29] Additionally, $PGD_2$ can induce bronchoconstriction through T prostanoid receptors, further contributing to the AERD phenotype.[29]

Recent studies suggest that CysLTs may induce the release of the structural cell-derived cytokines thymic stromal lymphopoietin (TSLP) and interleukin-33 (IL-33). TSLP can act directly on mast cells, promoting the release of mast-cell products, including $PGD_2$. TSLP and IL-33 are strongly expressed by nasal polypoid tissue in AERD.[29,36] Further, TSLP messenger RNA (mRNA) expression from nasal polypoid tissue in AERD correlates with urinary $PGD_2$ levels in these subjects.[37]

Cahill and colleagues[28] examined prostaglandin generation in patients with AERD undergoing therapeutic desensitization. They compared basal urinary prostaglandin metabolite and $LTE_4$ levels in patients with AERD before aspirin desensitization, after desensitization, and following 8 weeks of maintenance aspirin therapy with 1300 mg of aspirin per day. They found that daily aspirin therapy for 8 weeks led to a striking decrease in prostaglandin metabolite (M) levels as follows: PGE-M ($8.7 \pm 2.1$ pmol/mg Cr, $P<.01$), PGI-M ($0.14 \pm 0.03$ pmol/mg Cr, $P<.01$), TX-M ($0.2 \pm 0.1$ pmol/mg Cr, $P<.001$), and PGD-M ($2.2 \pm 0.8$ pmol/mg Cr, $P<.001$). In contrast, there was no change in $LTE_4$ levels ($2.7 \pm 1.2$ pmol/mg Cr, $P = .24$) (see **Fig. 2**). The authors postulate that the therapeutic benefit of high-dose aspirin in AERD may be, at least in part, the result of a reduction in these bronchoconstrictive prostaglandins. According to the investigators, the unexpected reduction in urinary PGE-M levels ($8.7 \pm 2.1$ pmol/mg Cr, $P<.01$) following 8 weeks of aspirin therapy may reflect the ability of high-dose aspirin to not only interfere with COX-1, but also to interfere with COX-2, which is responsible for most renal $PGE_2$ synthesis.

Interestingly, the subjects with AERD who were unable to tolerate aspirin challenge secondary to severe reactions not only demonstrated higher levels of CysLTs but also experienced a marked increase in urinary $PGD_2$, during their reaction, which correlated with the severity of airflow obstruction. In contrast, patients who were successfully desensitized and subsequently treated with high-dose aspirin displayed a steep reduction in urinary $PGD_2$ as well as an associated reduction in tissue eosinophils ($0.31 \pm 0.06$–$0.93 \pm 0.19$ $10^3/\mu L$, $P<.01$) and a modest reduction in tissue basophils. These data suggest that the aspirin therapy may lead to a reduction in $PGD_2$ generation, thereby precluding recruitment of $PGD_2$ responsive effector cells to the airways. Although the mechanism by which aspirin contributes to this decline has not been fully elucidated, it may be the result of aspirin-induced inhibition of IL-4 expression. As IL-4 is an activator of $PGD_2$ synthase, a reduction in IL-4 may subsequently lead to diminished production of $PGD_2$. The impact of aspirin therapy on IL-4 expression is discussed later in this article.

## DESENSITIZATION CHANGES IN CYSTEINYL LEUKOTRIENE RECEPTOR EXPRESSION

In 2002, Sousa and colleagues[19] examined the expression of $CysLT_1$ and $LTB_4$ receptors in inflammatory leukocytes from nasal biopsies of patients with AERD. Aspirin desensitization was associated with a significant reduction in cells expressing the $CysLT_1$ R, which was seen as early as 2 weeks and persisted through follow-up at 6 months. Although this finding may partially explain the clinical benefit of aspirin desensitization, the study did not postulate further as to why the $CysLT_1$ R was downregulated with continued aspirin therapy. As is discussed in the following section, this reduction in $CysLT_1$ R, expression likely results from aspirin-induced changes in IL-4 production.

## INTERLEUKIN-4 ALTERATIONS FOLLOWING ASPIRIN DESENSITIZATION

The cascade of inflammation in AERD involves the stimulatory signaling of various cytokines such as IL-5 promoting eosinophil development, differentiation, and survival, and IL-13–enhancing bronchial smooth muscle proliferation and inhibition of $PGE_2$ biosynthesis.[8] More recently, research has focused on the role of IL-4 in the development of AERD.

Hsieh and colleagues[32] studied the priming effects of IL-4 on the in vitro production of histamine, CysLTs, and PGs from human cord blood–derived MC. CysLT release was increased by 27-fold and $PGD_2$ release was increased by 6-fold when these MCs were passively stimulated with IL-4 in addition to stem cell factor (SCF). The addition of IL-3 or IL-5 to the 4/SCF-primed cells led to a further increase in CysLT production by sixfold and fourfold, respectively. This increase was found to occur as a result of IL-4 induction of $LTC_4$ S. Additional evidence published by Early and colleagues[38] showed the compounded effects of IL-4 on CysLT receptor expression. Using quantitative polymerase chain reaction (PCR) analysis of mRNA and receptor proteins extracted from immune cells, the investigators were able to show that IL-4 stimulation resulted in significant increases in both $CysLT_1R$ and $CysLT_2R$ on T and B lymphocytes ($P<.01$) and $CysLT_2R$ on eosinophils ($P<.05$). $CysLT_2R$ mRNA was also increased in monocytes, T cells, and B cells after IFN-$\gamma$ stimulation. The mechanisms of these effects have been shown to occur through IL-4/STAT6-dependent pathways, which are also important in the IL-4–induced suppression of PG production.[39–41] Combined results from these studies imply a likely role for IL-4 in the pathogenesis of AERD.

The pharmacologic effects of aspirin have been extended to include the inhibition of IL-4. Cianferoni and colleagues[26] examined the effect of aspirin on the expression of various cytokines, including IL-4, IL-13, IL-2, and IFN-$\gamma$ in purified human CD4$^+$ T cells. Experiments showed that therapeutic concentrations of aspirin significantly inhibited IL-4 secretion in peripheral blood T cells by $47\% \pm 2.4\%$ ($P<.05$) and that this inhibition occurred without significant aspirin-induced apoptosis to account for the change. Using multiple NSAIDs, the investigators showed that IL-4 suppression occurred independently of COX inhibition. They identified aspirin inhibition of IL-4 gene expression via salicylate-targeted regions in the IL-4 promoter as the possible mechanism of action, although the exact pathway was not defined. Aspirin did not have any significant effect on the levels of IL-2, IL-13, or IFN-$\gamma$ expression.

Expanding on these findings, several groups have now identified aspirin inhibition of IL-4–induced STAT6 activation as the possible mechanism associated with the therapeutic benefits of aspirin desensitization. Using a murine model, Perez and colleagues[42] showed that sodium salicylate (NaSal) and aspirin blocked the ability of IL-4 to induce DNA-binding activity of STAT6 in a dose-dependent manner (**Fig. 3**). They showed that aspirin inhibits IL-4–dependent induction of CD23 expression on human peripheral blood mononuclear cells. These findings were confirmed in a more recent study published by Steinke and colleagues.[27] Using THP-1 human mononuclear cells, they showed that aspirin inhibited IL-4–induced CysLT$_1$ R and F$_{c\epsilon}$ RI$_\alpha$ mRNA expression in a dose-dependent fashion. Similar results occurred with ketorolac but not NaSal. These investigators also reported the presence of STAT6-binding sites within the promoters for the CysLT $_1$ R and LTC $_4$ S, which are engaged by IL-4 nuclear extracts and were effectively inhibited by aspirin.

Katial and colleagues[21] reported the effects of aspirin desensitization on novel inflammatory sputum biomarkers in patients with AERD. In addition to IL-4, these investigators studied changes in sputum tryptase, matrix metallopeptidase 9 (MMP-9), tissue inhibitors of metalloproteinases 1 (TIMP-1) and FMS-like tyrosine kinase 3 ligand. Traditional measures such as symptom scores, exhaled nitric oxide (FeNO), and lung function were also assessed. Twenty-one patients were enrolled in the study,

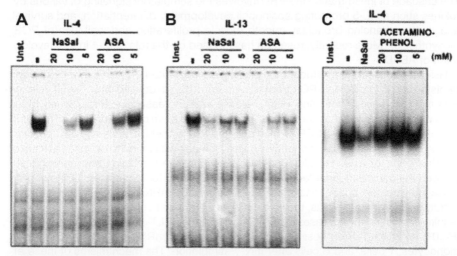

**Fig. 3.** Salicylates, but not acetaminophenol, inhibit STAT6 activation. (*A*) M12 cells were cultured with the indicated concentrations of NaSal and aspirin for 1 hour before stimulation with IL-4 (10 ng/mL) for 30 minutes. STAT6 DNA-binding activity in cell extracts was analyzed by electrophoretic mobility shift assay (EMSA) using the IFN-$\gamma$ activation site sequence contained in the C$\epsilon$ promoter. (*B*) U937 cells were cultured with NaSal or ASA for 1 hour, and then stimulated for 30 minutes with IL-13 (400 ng/mL). STAT6 activation was then analyzed by EMSA. (*C*) M12 cells were cultured with nothing, NaSal (20 mM), or the indicated concentrations of acetaminophenol. IL-4 was then added, and STAT6 binding to DNA was analyzed by EMSA. (*From* Perez-GM, Melo M, Keegan A, et al. Aspirin and salicylates inhibit the IL-4 and IL-13 induced activation of STAT6. J Immunol 2002;168:1429; with permission.)

with 16 completing successful sputum induction. Six months after desensitization, while on high-dose aspirin, sputum IL-4 levels decreased 94.7% (95% confidence interval [CI], 67%–99.2%) relative to baseline (baseline mean 28.1 pg/mL, 6-month mean 1.5 pg/mL; $P = .004$) (**Fig. 4**). This change was accompanied with a similar decrease in MMP-9 after 6 months. This suggests that the reported increases in CysLTs may be regulated by IL-4–dependent pathways, which are then downregulated by daily aspirin treatment after desensitization.

More recently, Katial and colleagues[43] investigated the mechanism underlying IL-4 suppression by aspirin therapy. They evaluated the in vitro effects of nonsteroidal anti-inflammatory drugs on the activation of peripheral blood CD4+ T cells through STAT6 signaling. Peripheral blood mononuclear cells from 11 aspirin-sensitive asthmatic individuals, 10 aspirin-tolerant asthmatic individuals, and 10 healthy controls were stimulated with anti-CD3 antibody and IL-4, both in the presence and absence of NSAIDs. Subsequently, the expression of phosphorylated STAT6 (pSTAT6), pSTAT4, and IL-4 were measured in CD4+ T lymphocytes by flow cytometry. They found that stimulation with the combination of anti-CD3 and IL-4 induced pSTAT6 in CD4+ T cells from all subjects; however, this induction was significantly higher in aspirin-sensitive asthmatic individuals as compared with controls. Aspirin, indomethacin, and to a lesser degree the weak COX-1 inhibitor sodium salicylate, inhibited pSTAT in all subjects in a dose-dependent manner (**Fig. 5**). These studies suggest that aspirin desensitization may be effective, in part, by the ability of COX-1 inhibitors to mitigate STAT6 signaling, thus blocking the biologic activities of IL-4 with subsequent downregulation of CysLT production and CysLT$_1$R expression.

## EFFECT OF ASPIRIN DESENSITIZATION ON LEUKOCYTE-DERIVED CYTOKINES

Studies addressing the cytokine milieu in AERD have demonstrated a predominantly $T_H2$-like profile, which is not surprising given the fundamental role of eosinophils in the

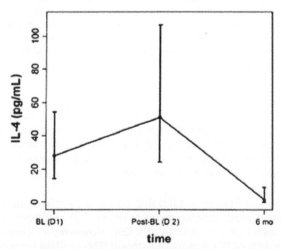

**Fig. 4.** IL-4 means over time, with 95% CIs, based on the linear mixed model fit. IL-4 was modeled on the natural log scale, and estimated and CI end points were then inverted back for presentation, resulting in longer upper bars than lower bars. Note that CIs are relevant for fixed time points only and do not indicate variability of estimated for differences between time points because repeated-measures data were involved. BL, baseline. (*From* Katial R, Strand M, Prasertsuntarasai T, et al. The effect of aspirin desensitization on novel biomarkers in aspirin-exacerbated respiratory diseases. J Allergy Clin Immunol 2010;126:741; with permission.)

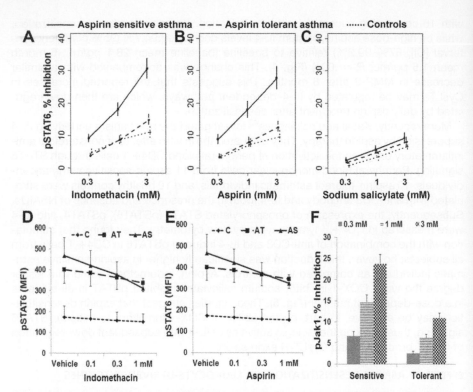

**Fig. 5.** (*A–F*) Comparison of the effect of indomethacin, aspirin, and sodium salicylate on CD4 T-cell pSTAT6 expression in aspirin-sensitive (n = 11) and aspirin-tolerant (n = 10) patients with asthma and control subjects (n = 10). (*F*) Effect of aspirin on phosphorylated Jak1 in aspirin-sensitive (n = 11) and aspirin-tolerant (n = 10) patients with asthma. $P = .01$ for 0.1 mM aspirin and $P<.01$ for other doses of aspirin (Mann-Whitney $U$ test). (*From* Katial RK, Martucci M, Burnett T et al. Nonsteroidal anti-inflammatory-induced inhibition of signal transducer and activator of transcription 6 (STAT-6) phosphorylation in aspirin-exacerbated respiratory disease. J Allergy Clin Immunol 2016;138(2):583; with permission.)

disease. However, newer observations suggest that AERD is characterized by a mixed $T_H1$ and $T_H2$ inflammatory profile with a prominent IFN-γ expression. Steinke and colleagues[44] highlighted this observation through their examination of the cytokine composition in nasal polyp tissue from subjects with AERD as compared with subjects with aspirin-tolerant chronic hyperplastic eosinophilic sinusitis (CHES) and healthy controls.

Through quantitative PCR of nasal polyp tissue, they found polyps from patients with AERD demonstrated variable expression of $T_H2$ cytokines and had significantly elevated levels of IL-4 mRNA ($P<.05$). However, in contrast to subjects with CHES, those with AERD also had profound IFN-γ mRNA transcript expression. They performed intracellular cytokine staining and reported that most of the IL-4 and IFN-γ staining was observed in eosinophils, indicating the eosinophilic source of these cytokines as well as their intracellular accumulation in the eosinophil granules.

Alteration of IFN-γ expression in T lymphocytes has also been reported in relation to aspirin desensitization. Shome and colleagues[45] demonstrated that subjects with

AERD have elevated baseline levels of IFN-$\gamma$ in circulating CD8+ T lymphocytes as compared with aspirin-tolerant controls. Interestingly, this pattern decreased significantly after desensitization, although neither the mechanism nor significance behind this change was elucidated.

## ROLE OF PLATELETS AND TARGETED ANTIPLATELET THERAPIES IN ASPIRIN-EXACERBATED RESPIRATORY DISEASE

There is relatively new evidence that the proinflammatory actions of activated platelets may play a central role in the pathogenesis of AERD. Increased membrane expression of P-selectin is a hallmark of platelet activation and mediates platelet adhesion to leukocytes through P-selectin glycoprotein ligand 1.[46] Platelet-leukocyte aggregates are well-recognized contributors to vascular inflammation and cardiovascular disease[47]; similarly, they may be effectors of AERD pathogenesis. Laidlaw and colleagues[48] found that peripheral blood and nasal polyp tissue from patients with AERD contained significantly more platelet-adherent leukocytes than aspirin-tolerant control subjects, and that 80% of the circulating eosinophils were adherent to platelets. Furthermore, these cells had increased expression of adhesion molecules such as beta integrins, implying that adherent platelets may facilitate adhesion and augment recruitment of eosinophils to peripheral tissue. An aberration in the process that controls this may contribute to the pathogenesis of AERD.

In response to activation, platelets precipitately liberate arachidonic acid from membrane lipids for conversion to eicosanoids such as $TXA_2$, which likewise facilitates leukocyte recruitment. $PGD_2$ is also generated, which signals through DP2 as a major chemoattractant for eosinophils, basophils, $T_H2$ cells, and innate type 2 helper cells. Thus, platelets are implicated as key mediators of leukocyte recruitment.[49]

In addition to self-generation of eicosanoids, platelets can also modulate the generation of leukotrienes by inflammatory leukocytes. Leukocytes can oxidize arachidonic acid through 5-LO to form $LTA_4$. Although neutrophils lack $LTC_4$ S activity and cannot convert $LTA_4$ into $LTC_4$, platelets possess abundant $LTC_4$ S activity in the absence of 5-LO.[50] In vitro studies have shown that neutrophils generate $LTA_4$ in excess of their ability to hydrolyze it to $LTB_4$; however, when platelets are added to the neutrophils, the excess $LTA_4$ is subsequently converted to $LTC_4$, suggesting that there is a reciprocal transcellular mechanism by which platelets might contribute to leukotriene generation, possibly by providing $LTC_4$ S.[48,51]

Supporting this theory, Laidlaw and colleagues[48] found that $uLTE_4$ levels strongly correlate with the percentage of platelet adherent leukocytes in the peripheral circulation. Additionally, $LTC_4$ S activity in blood granulocytes from patients with AERD was significantly higher than levels from aspirin-tolerant control subject granulocytes. Stripping the granulocytes of adherent platelets, resulted in a marked reduction in $LTC_4$ S activity, suggesting that adherent platelets likely contribute to CysLT overproduction in patients with AERD.

Indeed, aberrant platelet function may contribute to the pathogenesis of AERD and therapies which target platelet-leukocyte aggregates may represents a therapeutic option in these patients. Klinkhardt and colleagues[52] found that platelet-leukocyte aggregates are reduced by clopidogrel. It appears that 100 mg of daily aspirin does not reduce platelet-leukocyte aggregation, albeit this dose is likewise not sufficient to reduce nasal and pulmonary symptoms or prevent nasal polyp regrowth in AERD.[53] It may be that the high-dose aspirin required for the treatment AERD does result in platelet-leukocyte aggregate inhibition and contributes to the therapeutic benefit of aspirin therapy in these patients. This is an area in which further research is needed.

## SUMMARY

AERD is a clinical syndrome characterized by severe, persistent asthma, hyperplastic eosinophilic sinusitis with nasal polyps, and intolerance to aspirin and other NSAIDs that preferentially inhibit COX-1. Although aspirin desensitization has proved to be of significant long-term benefit in carefully selected patients with AERD, the mechanisms behind the therapeutic effects of aspirin desensitization have not been clearly delineated. Current research suggests that the derangements in inflammatory mediators seen in AERD may in part be a result of increased production and hyperresponsiveness to IL-4. This suggestion is reinforced by evidence that aspirin may derive its therapeutic benefit through direct inhibition of the IL-4–activated STAT6 pathway. The proposed mechanism would occur from continued aspirin ingestion causing inhibition of IL-4/STAT6–mediated production of CysLT and $CysLT_1$ R expression, with a subsequent attenuation of airway inflammation and clinical improvement (**Fig. 6**). Levels of $PGD_2$, a potent chemotactic for $T_H2$ cells, are also elevated at baseline in AERD and likely contribute to the eosinophilic airway inflammation characteristic of the disease. Interestingly, urinary $PGD_2$ levels decline following high-dose aspirin therapy, conceivably by preventing the chemotaxis of effector cells into the tissues.

Despite these advances, the limited data published regarding long-term mechanistic effects after aspirin desensitization leave many outstanding questions. Answering these questions requires further prospective, long-term evaluations of both the cellular and signaling alterations that occur in patients undergoing desensitization. In addition, as we learn more about the varied mechanisms of aspirin therapy related to inhibition of nuclear transcription factors, we may define new avenues of research exploration. Such further investigation will continue to increase our insight and understanding of this complex disease and it is hoped provide new therapeutic options and treatments for our patients.

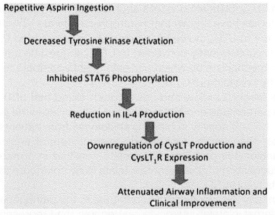

**Fig. 6.** Mechanism of inhibition of inflammation after aspirin desensitization. Proposed cascade of events after aspirin desensitization and continued ingestion. Signal inhibition via an IL-4/STAT6 pathway results in downregulation of CysLT production and $CysLT_1$ R expression, with subsequent reduction of tissue inflammation. (*From* Burnett T, Katial RK, Alam R. Mechanisms of aspirin desensitization. Immunol Allergy Clin North Am 2013;33(2):232; with permission.)

## REFERENCES

1. Vane J, Botting R. The mechanism of action of aspirin. Thromb Res 2003;110: 255–8.
2. Widal M, Abrami P, Lermeyez J. Anaphylaxieet idiosyncrasie. Presse Med 1922; 30:189–92.
3. Samter M, Beers R. Intolerance to aspirin: clinical studies and consideration of its pathogenesis. Ann Intern Med 1968;68:975–83.
4. Stevenson D, Simon RA, Mathison DA. Aspirin-sensitive asthma: tolerance to aspirin after positive oral aspirin challenges. J Allergy Clin Immunol 1980;66:82–8.
5. Stevenson D, Pleskow W, Simon R, et al. Aspirin-sensitive rhinosinusitis asthma: a double-blind cross-over study of treatment with aspirin. J Allergy Clin Immunol 1984;73:500–7.
6. Berges-Gimeno M, Simon R, Stevenson D. Early effects of aspirin desensitization treatment in asthmatic patients with aspirin-exacerbated respiratory disease. Ann Allergy Asthma Immunol 2003;90:338–41.
7. Berges-Gimeno M, Simon R, Stevenson D. Long-term treatment with aspirin desensitization in asthmatic patients with aspirin-exacerbated respiratory disease. J Allergy Clin Immunol 2003;111:180–6.
8. Farooque S, Lee T. Aspirin-sensitive respiratory disease. Annu Rev Physiol 2009; 71:465–87.
9. Szczeklik A, Stevenson D. Aspirin-induced asthma: advances in pathogenesis, diagnosis and management. J Allergy Clin Immunol 2003;111:913–21.
10. Stevenson D, Szczeklik A. Clinical and pathologic perspectives on aspirin sensitivity and asthma. J Allergy Clin Immunol 2006;118:773–86.
11. Szczeklik A, Sladek K, Dworski R, et al. Bronchial aspirin challenge causes specific eicosanoid response in aspirin-sensitive asthmatics. Am J Respir Crit Care Med 1996;154:1608–14.
12. Christie P, Tagari P, Ford-Hutchinson A, et al. Urinary leukotrienes $E_4$ concentrations increase after aspirin challenge in aspirin-sensitive asthmatic subjects. Am Rev Respir Dis 1991;143:1025–9.
13. Smith C, Hawksworth R, Thien F, et al. Urinary leukotrienes $E_4$ in bronchial asthma. Eur Respir J 1992;5:693–9.
14. Sladek K, Dworski R, Soja J, et al. Eicosanoids in bronchoalveolar lavage fluid of aspirin intolerant patients with asthma after aspirin challenge. Am J Respir Crit Care Med 1994;149:940–6.
15. Antczak A, Montuschi P, Kharitonov S, et al. Increased exhaled cysteinyl-leukotrienes and 8-isoprostane in aspirin-induced asthma. Am J Respir Crit Care Med 2001;166:301–6.
16. Picado C, Ramis I, Rosello J, et al. Release of peptide leukotrienes into nasal secretions after local instillation of aspirin in aspirin-sensitive asthmatic patients. Am Rev Respir Dis 1992;145:65–9.
17. Nasser S, Pfister R, Christie P, et al. Inflammatory cell populations in bronchial biopsies from aspirin-sensitive asthmatic subjects. Am J Respir Crit Care Med 1996;153:90–6.
18. Cowburn A, Sladek K, Soja J, et al. Overexpression of leukotrienes $C_4$ synthase in bronchial biopsies from patients with aspirin-intolerant asthma. J Clin Invest 1998; 101(4):834–6.
19. Sousa A, Parikh A, Scadding M, et al. Leukotriene-receptor expression on nasal mucosal inflammatory cells in aspirin-sensitive rhinosinusitis. N Engl J Med 2002; 347:1493–9.

20. Daffern P, Muilenburg D, Jugli T, et al. Association of urinary leukotriene $E_4$ excretion during aspirin challenges with severity of respiratory responses. J Allergy Clin Immunol 1999;104:559–64.
21. Katial R, Strand M, Prasertsuntarasai T, et al. The effect of aspirin desensitization on novel biomarkers in aspirin-exacerbated respiratory diseases. J Allergy Clin Immunol 2010;126:738–44.
22. Hamilos D, Leung D, Wood R, et al. Evidence for distinct cytokine expression in allergic versus nonallergic chronic sinusitis. J Allergy Clin Immunol 1995;96:537–44.
23. Riechelmann H, Deutschle T, Rozsasi A, et al. Nasal biomarker profiles in acute and chronic rhinosinusitis. Clin Exp Allergy 2005;35:1186–91.
24. Steinke J, Payne S, Borish L. Interleukin-4 in the generation of AERD phenotype: implications for molecular mechanisms driving therapeutic benefit of aspirin desensitization. J Allergy (Cairo) 2012;2012:182090.
25. Nasser S, Patel M, Bell G, et al. The effect of aspirin desensitization on urinary leukotriene $E_4$ concentrations in aspirin-sensitive asthma. Am J Respir Crit Care Med 1995;151:1326–30.
26. Cianferoni A, Schroeder J, Kim J, et al. Selective inhibition of interleukin-4 gene expression in human T cells by aspirin. Blood 2001;97:1742–9.
27. Steinke J, Culp J, Kropf E, et al. Modulation by aspirin of nuclear phospho-signal transducer and activator of transcription 6 expression: possible role in therapeutic benefit associated with aspirin desensitization. J Allergy Clin Immunol 2009; 124:724–30.
28. Cahill KN, Bensko JC, Boyce JA, et al. Prostaglandin D2: a dominant mediator of aspirin-exacerbated respiratory disease. J Allergy Clin Immunol 2015;135(1): 245–52.
29. Laidlaw TM, Boyce JA. Aspirin-exacerbated respiratory disease—new prime suspects. N Engl J Med 2016;374:484–8.
30. Lee T, Woszczek G, Farooque S. Leukotriene $E_4$: perspective on the forgotten mediator. J Allergy Clin Immunol 2009;124:417–21.
31. Arm J, O'Hickey S, Spur B, et al. Airway responsiveness to histamine and leukotriene E4 in subjects with aspirin-induced asthma. Am Rev Respir Dis 1989;140:148–53.
32. Hsieh F, Lam B, Penrose J, et al. T helper cell type 2 cytokines coordinately regulate immunoglobulin E-dependent cysteinyl leukotriene production by human cord blood-derived mast cells: profound induction of leukotriene C4 synthase expression by interleukin 4. J Exp Med 2001;193:123–33.
33. Juergens U, Christiansen M, Stevenson D, et al. Inhibition of monocyte leukotriene $B_4$ production after aspirin desensitization. J Allergy Clin Immunol 1995; 96:148–56.
34. Bochenek G, Nagraba K, Nizankowska E, et al. A controlled study of 9a,11b-PGF2 (a prostaglandin D2 metabolite) in plasma and urine of patients with bronchial asthma and healthy controls after aspirin challenge. J Allergy Clin Immunol 2003;111:743–9.
35. Hirai H, Tanaka K, Yoshie O, et al. Prostaglandin D2 selectively induces chemotaxis in T helper type 2 cells, eosinophils, and basophils via seven-transmembrane receptor CRTH2. J Exp Med 2001;193:255–61.
36. Liu T, Kanaoka Y, Barrett NA, et al. Aspirin-exacerbated respiratory disease involves a cysteinyl leukotriene-driven IL-33- mediated mast cell activation pathway. J Immunol 2015;195:3537–45.
37. Buchheit KM, Cahill KN, Katz HR. Thymic stromal lymphopoietin controls prostaglandin D2 generation in patients with aspirin-exacerbated respiratory disease. J Allergy Clin Immunol 2016;137(5):1566–76.e5.

38. Early S, Barekzi E, Negri J, et al. Concordant modulation of cysteinyl leukotriene receptor expression by IL-4 and IFN-γ on peripheral immune cells. Am J Respir Cell Mol Biol 2007;36:715–20.
39. Kaplan M, Wurster A, Smiley S, et al. STAT6-dependent and -independent pathways for IL-4 production. J Immunol 1999;163:6536–40.
40. Cho W, Kim Y, Jeoung D, et al. IL-4 and IL-13 suppress prostaglandins production in human follicular dendritic cells by repressing COX-2 and mPGES-1 expression through JAK1 and STAT6. Mol Immunol 2011;48:966–72.
41. Cho W, Jeoung D, Kim Y, et al. STAT6 and JAK1 are essential for IL-4 mediated suppression of prostaglandin production in human follicular dendritic cells: opposing roles of phosphorylated and unphosphorylated STAT6. Int Immunopharmacol 2012;12:635–42.
42. Perez GM, Melo M, Keegan A, et al. Aspirin and salicylates inhibit the IL-4 and IL-13 induced activation of STAT6. J Immunol 2002;168:1428–34.
43. Katial RK, Martucci M, Burnett T, et al. Non-steroidal antiinflammatory induced inhibition of STAT-6 phosphorylation in aspirin exacerbated respiratory disease. J Allergy Clin Immunol 2016. http://dx.doi.org/10.1016/j.jaci.2015.11.038.
44. Steinke JW, Liu L, Huyett P, et al. Prominent role of IFN-γ in patients with aspirin-exacerbated respiratory disease. J Allergy Clin Immunol 2013;132(4):856–65.
45. Shome GP, Tarbox J, Shearer M, et al. Cytokine expression in peripheral blood lymphocytes before and after aspirin desensitization in aspirin-exacerbated respiratory disease. Allergy Asthma Proc 2007;28:706–10.
46. Crovello CS, Furie BC, Furie B. Rapid phosphorylation and selective dephosphorylation of P-selectin accompanies platelet activation. J Biol Chem 1993;268:14590–3.
47. Totani L, Evangelista V. Platelet-leukocyte interactions in cardiovascular disease and beyond. Arterioscler Thromb Vasc Biol 2010;30(12):2357–61.
48. Laidlaw TM, Kidder MS, Bhattacharyya N, et al. Cysteinyl leukotriene overproduction in aspirin-exacerbated respiratory disease is driven by platelet-adherent leukocytes. Blood 2012;119:3790–8.
49. Laidlaw TM, Boyce JA. Platelets in patients with aspirin-exacerbated respiratory disease. J Allergy Clin Immunol 2015;135(6):1407–14.
50. Sala A, Zarini S, Folco G, et al. Differential metabolism of exogenous and endogenous arachidonic acid in human neutrophils. J Biol Chem 1999;274(40):28264–9.
51. Maclouf J, Antoine C, Henson PM, et al. Leukotriene C4 formation by transcellular biosynthesis. Ann N Y Acad Sci 1994;714:143–50.
52. Klinkhardt U, Bauersachs R, Adams J, et al. Clopidogrel but not aspirin reduces P-selectin expression and formation of platelet-leukocyte aggregates in patients with atherosclerotic vascular disease. Clin Pharmacol Ther 2003;73:232–41.
53. Rozsasi A, Polzehl D, Deutschle T, et al. Long-term treatment with aspirin desensitization: a prospective clinical trial comparing 100 and 300 mg aspirin daily. Allergy 2008;63(9):1228–34.

# Lipid Mediators in Aspirin-Exacerbated Respiratory Disease

Andrew R. Parker, MD, Andrew G. Ayars, MD,
Matthew C. Altman, MD, William R. Henderson Jr, MD*

## KEYWORDS

- AA (arachidonic acid) • AERD (aspirin-exacerbated respiratory disease) • Asthma
- COX (cyclooxygenase) • Leukotriene • 5-LO (5-lipoxygenase)
- NSAID (nonsteroidal inflammatory drug) • Prostaglandin

## KEY POINTS

- Patients with aspirin-exacerbated respiratory disease (AERD) have an anomalous underlying chronic inflammation characterized by mast cell and eosinophil infiltration/activation in the respiratory tract that is further exacerbated by nonsteroidal inflammatory drug (NSAID) ingestion.
- Dysregulation of arachidonic acid metabolism, both of the cyclooxygenase and 5-lipoxygenase pathways, is key to AERD pathogenesis.
- NSAID blockade of the bronchoprotective and antiinflammatory prostaglandin (PG) $E_2$ and resulting excessive production of the bronchoconstrictive and proinflammatory lipid mediators $PGD_2$ and cysteinyl leukotrienes $C_4$, $D_4$, and $E_4$ create a proallergic milieu in the airways of asthmatics with AERD.

## INTRODUCTION
### History

Aspirin-exacerbated respiratory disease (AERD) is a chronic inflammatory disorder of the respiratory tract characterized by the tetrad of asthma, nasal polyposis, rhinosinusitis, and acute exacerbations of the asthma and rhinosinusitis on ingestion of aspirin or other nonsteroidal antiinflammatory drugs (NSAIDs). Although reactions associated with the use of aspirin were described as early as 1902 by Hirschberg[1], just a few years after its synthesis, the entity of AERD was not described until 1922 by Widal and colleagues.[2] The clinical phenomenon of AERD was further delineated by Samter and Beers[3] in 1968 after they published a series of patients with asthma, nasal polyps,

Department of Medicine, UW Medicine, University of Washington, 750 Republican Street, Seattle, WA 98109-4766, USA
* Corresponding author.
E-mail address: wrhchem@uw.edu

Immunol Allergy Clin N Am 36 (2016) 749–763
http://dx.doi.org/10.1016/j.iac.2016.06.009          immunology.theclinics.com
0889-8561/16/$ – see front matter © 2016 Elsevier Inc. All rights reserved.

and aspirin sensitivity, and the entity became known as the Samter triad. The addition of chronic rhinosinusitis has since been recognized as a part of the clinical entity.[4] The disease has taken on several names in addition to Samter triad, including aspirin-induced asthma, aspirin-intolerant asthma, triad asthma, and aspirin hypersensitivity. There is now a preference for AERD because this is a more encompassing and accurate name; it indicates that this is an underlying respiratory tract disease that is exacerbated but not caused by NSAIDs. In 1971, Vane[5] published his discovery of the mechanism of action of aspirin, and, soon after, the capability of aspirin to inhibit the cyclooxygenase (COX) enzyme was implicated in the underlying pathogenesis of AERD, suggesting a dysregulation of arachidonic acid (AA) metabolism.[5,6] Although significant advancements in the understanding of the pathogenesis of AERD have been achieved since that time, in particular the skewing of the AA metabolic pathway to the overproduction of the 5-lipoxygenase (5-LO) products, the leukotriene (LT)s, much remains unknown about this disease of the upper and lower respiratory tract.

### Prevalence

The prevalence of AERD has been poorly understood because it is not always distinguished from other forms of asthma in the population. A recent meta-analysis of AERD prevalence among asthmatics examined 27 studies deemed appropriate out of 1770 articles on this topic and found a prevalence ranging from 5.5% to 12.4% with an estimated prevalence of 7.2% among all studies.[7] Patients with severe asthma had the highest prevalence of AERD at 14.9%, followed by patients with nasal polyps (9.7%) and chronic rhinosinusitis (8.7%).[7]

### Clinical Presentation

The disease typically presents in the second to fourth decade with chronic rhinitis and hyposmia.[8] The usual progression is subsequent development of sinusitis and nasal polyposis with a prominent eosinophilic infiltrate within months, and then symptoms typical of asthma within 1 to 2 years. Classically, such patients are sensitive to NSAIDs from the beginning of the manifestation of disease, and experience an exacerbation of symptoms with NSAID use in a dose-dependent fashion. Symptoms occur between 30 minutes to 3 hours after ingestion and can range from rhinitis to life-threatening bronchospasm. However, NSAID sensitivity may be noticed at any point in the disease depending on patient use of these medications. Although this is the classic presentation, atypical presentations are reported as well; most notably examples of patients with asthma who have tolerated NSAIDs in the past but become sensitive only later in the disease process.

### Pathophysiology

The cause of AERD is not known and the pathophysiology is only partially understood. Knowledge of the disease mechanism comes predominantly from observations showing differences that have been identified in individuals with AERD compared with aspirin-tolerant asthmatic individuals as well as nonasthmatics. From the time of disease onset, patients with AERD develop upper respiratory inflammation manifested as chronic rhinosinusitis with polyposis that progressively involves the lower respiratory tract in the form of persistent asthma. Although patients with AERD do have reactions after exposure to NSAIDs, with acute increases in inflammatory mediators after aspirin challenge, they also have baseline increases in airway inflammation compared with aspirin-tolerant controls.[9] Histologic evaluation has shown an increased density of eosinophils in the bronchial mucosa and submucosa as well as within the nasal mucosa and epithelium at baseline in biopsies from aspirin-sensitive, compared with aspirin-tolerant, asthmatics.[10,11] What drives this expansion of eosinophilic granulocytes is unclear. Levels of the eosinophil chemoattractant eotaxin-2 have been found to be increased at baseline and after aspirin challenge in aspirin-sensitive patients, but the perturbation that leads to increased levels of chemomediators in the first place is unknown.[12]

### Key Findings in Aspirin-exacerbated Respiratory Disease

The key findings in this disorder are as follows:

- Patients with AERD have an increased number of mast cells and eosinophils infiltrating the respiratory mucosa, even in the absence of NSAID exposure.[13]
- There is an increase in numerous cytokines known to recruit mast cells and eosinophils including interleukin (IL)-3, IL-4, IL-5, IL-13, granulocyte-macrophage colony-stimulating factor, and eotaxin in bronchoalveolar lavage (BAL) fluid and respiratory tissue.[14]
- There is an increase in the 5-LO products of AA metabolism (ie, the cysteinyl leukotriene [CysLT]s $LTC_4$, $LTD_4$, and $LTE_4$, which each contain the amino acid cysteine bound to their lipid structure) and other proinflammatory lipid mediators in BAL fluid.[15]
- There is an increase in CysLT receptors in the upper and lower respiratory mucosa.[16]
- There is an increase in the $LTC_4$ synthase enzyme.[17]
- There is a decrease in levels of lipoxins.[18]
- There is alteration in the formation of the COX AA products, with a decrease in prostaglandin (PG)$E_2$ and increase in $PGD_2$.[14]

These findings implicate abnormal AA metabolism and altered sensitivity to the downstream lipid mediators as the primary driving force behind the clinical manifestations of AERD. Mast cell and eosinophil activation and production of AA metabolites likely play a dominant role in AERD pathophysiology. Arachidonate metabolism is complex and results in numerous lipid mediators that can be either proinflammatory, antiinflammatory, or have mixed effects depending on the target receptors.

## ROLE OF CYCLOOXYGENASE ARACHIDONIC ACID METABOLISM IN ASPIRIN-EXACERBATED RESPIRATORY DISEASE
### Prostaglandin Synthesis

Prostanoids are a subclass of eicosanoids that include prostaglandins, thromboxanes, and prostacyclins and are potent pro and antiinflammatory mediators. They can have vastly different effects depending on the receptor involved, cellular context, and signal transduction pathways.[19] These agents are known to play a role in inflammation, platelet aggregation, and vasodilation/vasoconstriction, among other effects. Prostaglandins were discovered by the Swedish pharmacologist Ulf von Euler in 1935 after being isolated in semen. It was thought that prostaglandins originated from the prostate, which is how the name originated. Although prostaglandins are generally thought to be proinflammatory, some of these mediators have antiinflammatory effects depending on factors such as production location and specific receptor and signaling pathways. The prostanoids include $PGD_2$, $PGE_2$, $PGF_2$, $PGI_2$ (prostacyclin), and thromboxane (TX) $A_2$ (**Fig. 1**).

The synthesis of prostanoids involves a multistep sequence, the first of which is hydrolysis of AA by cytosolic phospholipase (cPL)$A_2$ and secretory phospholipase (sPL) $A_2$s (see **Fig. 1**).[20–22] These steps involve the oxygenation of AA by COX-1 and COX-2

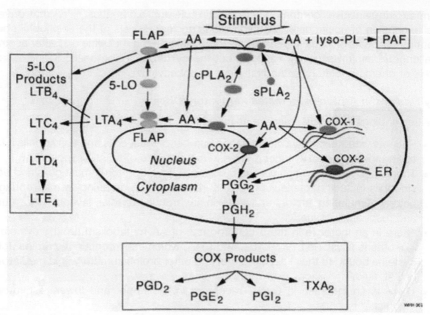

**Fig. 1.** 5-LO and COX products of AA metabolism. Fundamental to AA metabolism are the COX-1 and COX-2 and the 5-LO enzymes. AA, the precursor to all leukotriene and prostaglandin products, is released from the glycerol backbones of cellular membrane phospholipids by the action of cytosolic phospholipase $A_2$ ($cPLA_2$) and secretory phospholipase $A_2$ ($sPLA_2$). This process occurs in inflammatory cells by the action of various stimuli, such as allergen crosslinking of immunoglobulin E (IgE) bound to high-affinity IgE receptors in mast cells. COX-1 acts on AA to yield prostaglandins and/or thromboxanes. In mast cells, $PGG_2$ is the first chemical intermediate formed that can be converted to the potent antiinflammatory mediator $PGE_2$. These mediators act on bronchiole smooth muscle with bronchodilatory effects, and also inhibit proinflammatory metabolic pathways. In particular, $PGE_2$ is a potent inhibitor of the 5-LO enzyme. Of note, this pathway also generates $PGD_2$, a potent bronchoconstrictor that counteracts the effects of $PGE_2$. (*Adapted from* Chilton FH, Fonteh AN, Surette ME, et al. Control of arachidonate levels within inflammatory cells. Biochim Biophys Acta 1996;1299(1):11; with permission.)

(also known as prostaglandin endoperoxide H synthases 1 and 2), yielding $PGG_2$ and then $PGH_2$. $PGH_2$ is subsequently converted to $PGD_2$, $PGE_2$, $PGF_2$, $PGI_2$, or $TxA_2$ via specific synthases.[23] Prostanoid receptors include the $PGD_2$ receptors 1 ($DP_1$) and 2 ($DP_2$, also called CRTH2 [chemoattractant receptor homologue expressed by type 2 helper T cells]), PGE receptors 1, 2, 3, and 4 (i.e., $EP_1$, $EP_2$, $EP_3$, and $EP_4$), $PGF_2$ receptor (FP), $PGI_2$ receptor (IP), and $TXA_2$ receptor (TP). In the lungs, $PGE_2$ provides an antiinflammatory and bronchoprotective effect, whereas $PGD_2$ has been shown to exert both proinflammatory and bronchoconstrictor effects. The altered formation of $PGE_2$ relative to $PGD_2$ in the airways of patients with AERD is a prominent feature of this disorder.

## Prostaglandin $E_2$

Most of the data in asthma, and specifically AERD, highlight the antiinflammatory effects of $PGE_2$ acting through the $EP_2$ receptor. $PGE_2$ is an important cofactor in regulating the production of CysLTs, blocking activation of 5-LO in leukocytes.[24–26] Lung mast cell degranulation is also inhibited by $PGE_2$ in an $EP_2$-depended manner.[27] Knockout mice deficient in $PGE_2$ synthase and unable to generate $PGE_2$ have an AERD-like phenotype showing increased airway hyperresponsiveness, mast cell activation, and CysLT production when challenged with aspirin.[28]

In the human lung, $PGE_2$ has been shown to relax the bronchi through the $EP_2$ receptor precontracted by histamine.[29] In bronchial biopsies, patients with AERD have reduced percentages of T cells, macrophages, mast cells, and neutrophils expressing the $EP_2$ receptor compared with aspirin-tolerant asthmatics and normal controls. In vitro $PGE_2$ inhibits cytokine production by peripheral blood mononuclear cells through $EP_2$.[30] The bronchial fibroblasts of patients with asthma, and specifically AERD, produce less $PGE_2$ after stimulation compared with normal controls.[31] Inhaled $PGE_2$ prevents the bronchoconstriction associated with bronchial challenge in patients with aspirin-tolerant asthma after allergen challenge as well as in patients with AERD challenged with lysine acetylsalicylate.[32,33]

Fibroblasts from nasal polyps of control subjects produce increased levels of $PGE_2$ when exposed to IL-1$\beta$, whereas the fibroblasts from patients with AERD do not.[34] The nasal polyps of patients with AERD have a higher frequency of extravascular platelets and peripheral blood contained higher percentages of circulating neutrophils, eosinophils, and monocytes with adherent platelets. This finding is thought to be important because these platelets contribute $LTC_4$ synthase with increased production of CysLTs, as described later.[35]

Leukocytes from patients with AERD release more CysLTs following aspirin stimulation compared with patients with asthma without aspirin sensitivity and normal controls; when $PGE_2$ is added to these leukocytes in vitro, the levels of CysLTs decrease, indicating an inhibitory effect of $PGE_2$.[36] Percentages of neutrophils; mast cells; eosinophils; and T cells expressing EP1, EP3, and EP4 are significantly reduced in patients with AERD compared with aspirin-tolerant asthmatics.[37]

### Prostaglandin $D_2$

Although $PGE_2$ is known to have antiinflammatory effects in the lungs, $PGD_2$ has direct inflammatory effects in the lungs of asthmatics, including patients with AERD. $PGD_2$ recruits inflammatory cells, including basophils, eosinophils, Th2 cells, and type 2 innate lymphoid cells through $DP_1$ and $DP_2$.[38] In mice deficient in the $PGD_2$ receptor $DP_1$, the concentrations of proallergic Th2 cytokines and the extent of lymphocyte accumulation in the lung are greatly reduced compared with those in wild-type animals after challenge.[39] In nasal polyp tissue, the $PGD_2/PGE_2$ ratio is highest in the nasal polyp tissue of patients with AERD.[40] In the lungs, baseline sputum levels of $PGD_2$ are higher in patients with AERD compared with aspirin-tolerant asthmatics without differences in baseline $PGE_2$.[41] After lysyl-aspirin challenge there occurs a significant decline in $PGE_2$ levels accompanied by an increase in levels of CysLTs $LTD_4$ and $LTE_4$ in patients with AERD.

Analyzing systemic production, patients with AERD have higher plasma levels of baseline $PGD_2$ as well as an increase in mast cell tryptase levels at baseline compared with aspirin-tolerant asthmatics and controls.[42] Higher urinary levels of $PGD_2$ are found in patients with AERD compared with controls and these levels increase further during reactions to aspirin. This spike in $PGD_2$ levels during reactions also correlates with a reduction in eosinophil levels that may be caused by migration of eosinophils into the tissues during an exacerbation. A clinical trial (NCT02216357, ClinicalTrials. gov) to determine the safety and potential clinical benefit of the TP receptor antagonist ifetroban in patients with AERD has recently been completed. Baseline levels of urinary $PGE_2$ are similar in aspirin-tolerant patients compared with patients with

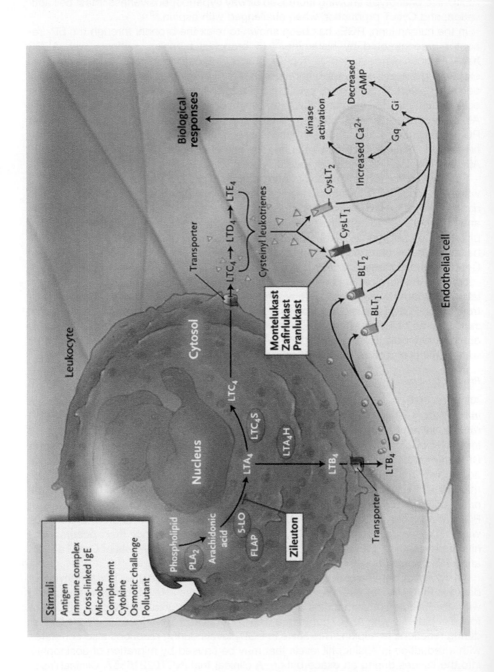

AERD.[43,44] When challenged with the selective COX2 inhibitor celecoxib, both patients with AERD and aspirin-tolerant asthmatics show a decrease in $PGE_2$ levels.[43,44]

Several aspirin desensitization procedures have been developed and are based on escalating doses of aspirin followed by daily exposure to maintain desensitization. The desensitized patients have decreases in nasal congestion, need for surgery, and steroid use acutely; and, chronically, they have decrease in infectious sinusitis together with improvement in sense of smell and asthma control.[45] Patients who undergo aspirin desensitization and continue on high-dose aspirin therapy have decreased levels of urinary $PGD_2$ and increased levels of peripheral eosinophils; this may be caused by the decrease in recruitment caused by the chemoattractant nature of $PGD_2$.[46] The urinary levels of $PGE_2$ also decrease after 8 weeks of high-dose aspirin desensitization. Patients unable to complete their desensitization protocols because of adverse reactions such as cutaneous and gastrointestinal manifestations had significant increases in basal $PGD_2$ level.[46]

## ROLE OF 5-LIPOXYGENASE ARACHIDONIC ACID METABOLISM IN ASPIRIN-EXACERBATED RESPIRATORY DISEASE
### Leukotriene Synthesis

Once AA is liberated by phospholipases $A_2$ ($PLA_2$s) (**Fig. 2**), it is converted by 5-LO in the presence of 5-LO–activating protein (FLAP) to 5-hydroperoxyeicosatetraenoic acid (5-HPETE), which is the branch point for production of either leukotrienes via production of $LTA_4$ by the same 5-LO enzyme, or else lipoxins by alternative lipoxygenase enzymes. $LTA_4$ is a temporary intermediate that is rapidly converted to $LTB_4$ by $LTA_4$ hydrolase ($LTA_4H$) or to $LTC_4$ after conjugation with reduced glutathione by leukotriene $C_4$ synthase ($LTC_4S$) (see **Fig. 2**). In a process termed transcellular biosynthesis, cells like platelets and endothelial cells that lack sufficient 5-LO or FLAP to produce leukotrienes by themselves are able to take up $LTA_4$ derived from leukocytes and form leukotrienes because they have the downstream enzymes $LTA_4H$ or $LTC_4S$. One example of this process is the interaction between platelets and leukocytes, which may contribute to leukotriene overproduction in patients with AERD as follows: neutrophils are unable to form $LTC_4$ because they lack $LTC_4S$ and platelets lack 5-LO but do contain $LTC_4S$; in a P-selectin–dependent interaction, platelets adherent to the leukocytes can convert neutrophil-derived $LTA_4$ to $LTC_4$.[47]

---

**Fig. 2.** Generation of LTs and LT receptor–mediated signaling. A variety of stimuli, including antigen, immune complexes, complement, cytokines, and environmental pollutants, trigger leukotriene synthesis by activation of $PLA_2$s that catalyze AA hydrolysis from membrane phospholipids. 5-LO and FLAP present near the perinuclear membrane and convert AA to $LTA_4$. Leukotriene synthesis is blocked by the 5-LO inhibitor zileuton. $LTA_4H$ and $LTC_4S$ respectively act on $LTA_4$ to form $LTB_4$ and $LTC_4$, which are transferred out of the cytosol by carrier proteins. $LTC_4$ is then rapidly metabolized to $LTD_4$ and $LTD_4$ to $LTE_4$ extracellularly. $LTB_4$ and the CysLTs (ie, $LTC_4$, $LTD_4$, $LTE_4$) exert their biological effects through their engagement of cognate receptors on target cells. $LTB_4$ acts on its high-affinity receptor B leukotriene receptor 1 ($BLT_1$) on leukocytes and its lower affinity receptor B leukotriene receptor 2 ($BLT_2$), which is found more broadly. The CysLTs act on 2 receptors, CysLT receptor 1 ($CysLT_1$) and CysLT receptor 2 ($CysLT_2$), which are widely expressed. Montelukast, pranlukast, and zafirlukast are specific $CysLT_1$ receptor antagonist drugs. Activation of the Gq class of G proteins by these leukotriene receptors also increases levels of the Gi class and intracellular calcium, leading to a decrease in intracellular cyclic AMP (cAMP) levels and subsequent protein kinase activation to mediate the biological response in the target cells. (*From* Peters-Golden M, Henderson WR. Leukotrienes. N Engl J Med 2007;357:1843; with permission.)

Specific transporter proteins export $LTB_4$ and $LTC_4$ outside the cell (see **Fig. 2**). Extracellular sequential amino acid hydrolysis converts $LTC_4$ to leukotriene $LTD_4$ and then to $LTE_4$, which is the stable, active end metabolite. Lipoxins including lipoxin $A_4$ ($LXA_4$) and lipoxin $B_4$ ($LXB_4$) generally counterbalance the leukotrienes by antagonistic effects at the leukotriene receptors.[8]

### Increased Cysteinyl Leukotriene Production in Aspirin-exacerbated Respiratory Disease

The balance of AA metabolites is perturbed in AERD with a shift toward proinflammatory mediators, in particular the CysLTs. The imbalance of $PGE_2$ (decreased) and $PGD_2$ (increased) has the dual effect of increasing bronchoconstriction and decreasing inhibition of leukotriene production. Similarly, the imbalance of CysLTs (increased $LTC_4$, $LTD_4$, and $LTE_4$ levels) relative to lipoxins (decreased) leads to a proinflammatory state. Numerous studies have implicated the importance of increased production of leukotrienes, in particular CysLTs, in AERD pathophysiology. Initial studies showed that baseline levels of urinary $LTE_4$ excretion, a measure of leukotriene synthesis, was 6 times greater in aspirin-sensitive versus aspirin-tolerant asthmatics.[48] Furthermore, on aspirin challenge, the baseline level of $LTE_4$ excretion increased remarkably in the aspirin-sensitive group, whereas the aspirin-tolerant group remained at their prechallenge levels.[48] This finding suggests that CysLT overproduction is a key component in AERD. In contrast, no increase in $LTB_4$ has been found in either BAL fluid or nasal secretions in patients with AERD.[15,49]

$LTC_4S$ is expressed at 5 times greater levels in bronchial tissue biopsies from patients with aspirin-exacerbated asthma compared with biopsies from patients with aspirin-tolerant asthma, and 18 times more than in biopsies from individuals without asthma.[10] Of note, other associated enzymes in the AA metabolic pathway, including FLAP, 5-LO, $LTA_4$ hydrolase, COX-1, and COX-2, are expressed similarly between the 3 groups. A 4-fold greater expression of $LTC_4S$ and 3-fold greater expression of 5-LO is seen in the nasal mucosal eosinophilic infiltration of aspirin-intolerant patients compared with aspirin-tolerant patients; the increased enzymatic expression is likely caused by increased presence of eosinophils in aspirin-intolerant patients rather than increased expression of this enzyme by individual cells.[11] Although the development and persistence of AERD is thought to be mediated through multiple abnormalities within the leukotriene/prostaglandin cascade, these studies have been unable to determine whether increased $LTC_4S$ expression and CysLT production are causal in the development of AERD or are effects of increased airway inflammation with other inciting causes. In transgenic mice with overexpression of $LTC_4S$, the increased levels of CysLT that occur on NSAID challenge with sulpyrine are associated with a subsequent increase in airway inflammation similar to an AERD-like phenotype.[50] These data suggest that CysLT overproduction may be a primary factor in the development of AERD.[50]

Platelet-leukocyte interactions may contribute to the overproduction of CysLTs in patients with AERD. Nasal polyps from patients with AERD have platelets colocalized with leukocytes in these tissues and peripheral blood leukocytes from these individuals with AERD have more eosinophils, neutrophils, and monocytes in the blood with adherent platelets than are found in controls without AERD.[35] In the patients with AERD, the increased urinary $LTE_4$ levels observed correlated with the number of platelet-adherent leukocytes in the circulation.[35] Prasugrel, which blocks the purinergic receptor P2Y12 adenosine diphosphate (ADP)–mediated platelet activation and aggregation, is now being investigated for therapeutic benefit in patients with AERD (NCT01597375, ClinicalTrials.gov). Nasal polyps from patients with AERD also have increased expression of IL-33 and thymic stromal lymphopoietin, which promote eosinophilic inflammation in the airways.[51] Mouse models of AERD have been used to show the importance of CysLTs in IL-33–induced airway bronchoconstriction and mast cell activation and the eosinophilic inflammatory response.[51,52]

## BIOLOGICAL EFFECTS OF LEUKOTRIENES AND RECEPTOR-MEDIATED SIGNALING

The biological effects of leukotrienes are mediated through a variety of G-protein–coupled receptors of the rhodopsin class (**Box 1**; see **Fig. 2**). On leukotriene binding, a conformational change in the receptor protein communicates a transmembrane signal that results in increased intracellular calcium levels and reduced cyclic AMP levels. Downstream kinase cascades are then initiated, which result in the biological effects.

### Leukotriene $B_4$ Receptors

The effects of $LTB_4$ are mediated through the $BLT_1$ and $BLT_2$ receptors. $BLT_1$ is a high-affinity receptor for $LTB_4$. This receptor is primarily expressed on activated leukocytes and to a lesser extent in the spleen and thymus.[53] On activation, the $BLT_1$ receptor

---

**Box 1**
**Biological effects of leukotrienes on the actions of cells**

*Dendritic cells*

- Activation[a]
- Trafficking[a]

*Endothelial cells*

- Angiogenesis[a]
- Vascular permeability[a]

*Epithelial cells*

- Airway mucus release[a]
- Goblet cell numbers[a]

*Fibroblasts/myofibroblasts*

- Collagen release[a]
- Proliferation[a]

*Leukocytes*

- Activation/recruitment of airway mast cells[b], eosinophils[c], monocytes[b], T cells[c]
- Adhesion molecule expression[c]
- Cytokine/chemokine production[c]
- Reactive $O_2$ species generation[c]
- Type 2 helper T-cell (Th2) responses[c]

*Smooth muscle cells*

- Contractility[a]
- Proliferation[a]

   [a] Biological actions most characteristic of CysLTs.
   [b] Biological actions most characteristic of $LTB_4$.
   [c] Biological actions most characteristic of both CysLTs and $LTB_4$.
   (*Adapted from* Peters-Golden M, Henderson WR. Leukotrienes. N Engl J Med 2007;357:1846; with permission.)

---

promotes leukocyte attraction as well as adhesion of leukocytes to vascular endothelial cells. The other receptor, $BLT_2$, has lower affinity for $LTB_4$ but also recognizes other 5-LO products of AA metabolism, such as 5-HPETE. $BLT_2$ is expressed more widely than $BLT_1$, primarily in the spleen but also in the liver, ovary, and white blood cells.[53] The biological effects of $BLT_2$ seem to be diverse and are actively being investigated.

### Cysteinyl Leukotriene Receptors

The CysLTs exert their effect through the G-protein–coupled receptors $CysLT_1$ and $CysLT_2$.[54] $CysLT_1$ has the highest affinity for $LTD_4$ followed by $LTC_4$ and $LTE_4$ based on in vitro studies. In contrast, CysLT2 has fairly equal affinity for $LTC_4$ and $LTD_4$, with lesser affinity for $LTE_4$.[55] $CysLT_1$ is widely expressed on bronchial smooth muscle cells, eosinophils, mast cells, and neutrophils, as well as in the spleen, lung, and small intestine. $CysLT_1$ receptor expression can be upregulated by Th2-type cytokines, including IL-4, IL-5, and IL-13.[56] On activation, $CysLT_1$ results in bronchoconstriction and increased vascular permeability (see **Box 1**). In patients with persistent asthma, such as AERD, the CysLTs are major mediators of airway thickening and remodeling by stimulating fibroblast/myofibroblast and goblet cell proliferation, leading to excess collagen and mucus release respectively. $LTB_4$ and the CysLTs also promote Th2 cytokine and chemokine responses in leukocytes infiltrating the airways, amplifying the asthmatic response.

The $CysLT_1$ receptor pathway has been implicated in the pathophysiology of aspirin-sensitive asthma. Despite aspirin-sensitive and aspirin-tolerant asthmatics having the same number of leukocytes in their nasal mucosa, the percentage of those leukocytes expressing $CysLT_1$ is significantly greater in the aspirin-sensitive patients.[16] Moreover, aspirin desensitization in the aspirin-sensitive group results in the decreased expression of $CysLT_1$ within 2 weeks of desensitization.[16] $CysLT_2$ is expressed on similar cells as $CysLT_1$.

Although it is well established that the effects of both $LTC_4$ and $LTD_4$ are mediated through $CysLT_1$ and $CysLT_2$, the primary receptor for $LTE_4$ has been less clear. $LTE_4$, the most stable of the CysLTs, was recognized to be a powerful mediator of bronchoconstriction, nearly 40 times more potent than histamine in patients with asthma. $LTE_4$ induces infiltration by eosinophils and neutrophils (eosinophils 10 times greater than neutrophils) of the airway lamina propria after inhalation into the lungs of asthmatics.[57] However, initial studies showed its low affinity for $CysLT_1$ and $CysLT_2$ binding in vitro.[58,59] Later experiments using $CysLT_1$ and $CysLT_2$ knockout mice concluded that other receptors are likely involved in the activity of $LTE_4$ because increased vascular permeability was observed after $LTE_4$ exposure despite the lack of CysLT receptors.[60] Since that time, studies have indicated that P2Y12 and peroxisome proliferator-activated receptor gamma (PPARγ) receptors as well as the G-protein–coupled receptor 99 (GPR99), which has homology to the $P2Y_1$ nucleotide receptor subfamily, may be involved in $LTE_4$ signaling.[61–63] Mice deficient in GPR99 fail to release epithelial cell mucin in response to $LTE_4$, indicating an important role for this receptor in airway epithelial cell function.[64] Recent studies using a murine model suggest that $LTE_4$ signals more robustly than was previously thought through the $CysLT_1$ receptor, resulting in sustained phosphorylation and therefore greater in vivo effect than was suggested by the prior in vitro receptor affinity studies.[65]

## LEUKOTRIENES ANTAGONISTS IN THE TREATMENT OF ASPIRIN-EXACERBATED RESPIRATORY DISEASE

Treatment of AERD includes the same treatment options that exist for other forms of asthma, including beta-2 agonists, corticosteroids, and anticholinergics. However, in addition, leukotriene synthesis inhibitors and leukotriene receptor antagonists have been shown to be particularly effective in AERD and should be a primary therapy in the management of AERD. Given the role of leukotrienes in asthma, several compounds have been developed to interrupt this inflammatory pathway, and are collectively known as leukotriene-modifier drugs.

### 5-Lipoxygenase Inhibitors

Zileuton, a 5-LO inhibitor (see **Fig. 2**), was shown to reduce baseline and post–aspirin challenge urinary levels of $LTE_4$ in subjects with AERD.[66] This same study showed that zileuton also blunted the effects on forced expiratory volume in 1 second after aspirin challenge and mitigated the nasal and gastrointestinal symptoms associated with NSAID administration.[66] Although zileuton was promising given its ability to reduce the production of CysLTs as well as $LTB_4$, its clinical utility has been variable, likely because of its failure to completely block LT formation. Other studies have shown that although zileuton can increase the threshold dose of aspirin required to provoke a reaction, the effect of 5-LO inhibition can be overcome.[67] The widespread use of zileuton has been complicated by hepatotoxicity and the need for frequent dosing.

### Cysteinyl Leukotriene 1 Receptor Antagonists

Drugs developed to counter the effects of CysLTs are the $CysLT_1$ receptor antagonists (see **Fig. 2**). Montelukast, the most common of this class of medications in the United States, has been evaluated in the treatment of AERD. Much like zileuton, montelukast was shown to reduce, but not eliminate, reactions in a dose-dependent manner on aspirin challenge.[68] Although reactions after aspirin administration are not eliminated, montelukast reduces bronchospasm and shifts the upper and lower respiratory tract responses to the upper tract alone on NSAID challenge.[69] The upper airway effects, consisting of congestion, rhinorrhea, sneezing, and ocular symptoms, are likely secondary to the effects of other inflammatory mediators like histamine that are released by activated mast cells in the AERD nasal mucosa.

### SUMMARY

The predominant disorders in AERD include a chronic overproduction of proinflammatory leukotrienes as well as an increased sensitivity to their actions. These disorders result in recruitment of mast cells and eosinophils to the respiratory mucosa, and activation of these cells, which in turn increase leukotriene production further. This perturbed proinflammatory state results in the chronic rhinitis, asthma, and nasal polyps that characterize the disease. This disorder is acutely exacerbated by NSAIDs, namely through selective blockade of COX-1. Inhibition of this enzyme acutely blocks $PGE_2$ production and so further increases leukotriene levels. Although this has not been proved, it is the widely accepted mechanism and is supported by the fact that the COX-2 inhibitors do not lead to symptoms. This NSAID sensitivity is what clinically distinguishes patients with AERD from other asthmatics. Further research will be important to better understand the pathophysiology of this disease in which lipid mediators play such an important role.

### REFERENCES

1. Hirschberg A. Mitteilung über einen Fall von Nebenwirkungen des Aspirin. Dtsch Med Wschr 1902;28:416–7.
2. Widal MF, Abrami P, Lermeyez J. Anaphylaxie et idosyncrasie. Presse Med 1922; 30:189–92.

3. Samter M, Beers RF. Intolerance to aspirin. Clinical studies and consideration of its pathogenesis. Ann Intern Med 1968;68(5):975–83.

4. Borrish L. Sinusitis and asthma: entering the realm of evidence-based medicine. J Allergy Clin Immunol 2002;109(4):606–8.

5. Vane JR. Inhibition of prostaglandin synthesis as a mechanism of action for aspirin-like drugs. Nat New Biol 1971;231(25):232–5.

6. Szczeklik A, Gryglewski RJ, Czerniawska-Mysik G. Relationship of inhibition of prostaglandin biosynthesis by analgesics to asthma attacks in aspirin-sensitive patients. Br Med J 1975;1(5949):67–9.

7. Rajan JP, Wineinger NE, Stevenson DD, et al. Prevalence of aspirin-exacerbated respiratory disease among asthmatic patients: a meta-analysis of the literature. J Allergy Clin Immunol 2015;135(3):676–81.e1.

8. Stevenson DD, Zuraw BL. Pathogenesis of aspirin-exacerbated respiratory disease. Clin Rev Allergy Immunol 2003;24(2):169–88.

9. Gaber F, Daham K, Higashi A, et al. Increased levels of cysteinyl-leukotrienes in saliva, induced sputum, urine and blood from patients with aspirin-intolerant asthma. Thorax 2008;63(12):1076–82.

10. Cowburn AS, Sladek K, Soja J, et al. Overexpression of leukotriene $C_4$ synthase in bronchial biopsies from patients with aspirin-intolerant asthma. J Clin Invest 1998; 101(4):834–46.

11. Adamjee J, Suh Y-J, Park H-S, et al. Expression of 5-lipoxygenase and cyclooxygenase pathway enzymes in nasal polyps of patients with aspirin-intolerant asthma. J Pathol 2006;209(3):392–9.

12. Makowska JS, Grzegorczyk J, Bienkiewicz B, et al. Systemic responses after bronchial aspirin challenge in sensitive patients with asthma. J Allergy Clin Immunol 2008;121(2):348–54.

13. Yamashita T, Tsuji H, Maeda N, et al. Etiology of nasal polyps associated with aspirin-sensitive asthma. Rhinol Suppl 1989;8:15–24.

14. Stevenson DD, Szczeklik A. Clinical and pathologic perspectives on aspirin sensitivity and asthma. J Allergy Clin Immunol 2006;118(4):773–86 [quiz: 787–8].

15. Sladek K, Dworski R, Soja J, et al. Eicosanoids in bronchoalveolar lavage fluid of aspirin-intolerant patients with asthma after aspirin challenge. Am J Respir Crit Care Med 1994;149(4 Pt 1):940–6.

16. Sousa AR, Parikh A, Scadding G, et al. Leukotriene-receptor expression on nasal mucosal inflammatory cells in aspirin-sensitive rhinosinusitis. N Engl J Med 2002; 347(19):1493–9.

17. Weller CL, Collington SJ, Brown JK, et al. Leukotriene $B_4$, an activation product of mast cells, is a chemoattractant for their progenitors. J Exp Med 2005;201(12): 1961–71.

18. Sanak M, Levy BD, Clish CB, et al. Aspirin-tolerant asthmatics generate more lipoxins than aspirin-intolerant asthmatics. Eur Respir J 2000;16(1):44–9.

19. Hata AN, Breyer RM. Pharmacology and signaling of prostaglandin receptors: multiple roles in inflammation and immune modulation. Pharmacol Ther 2004; 103(2):147–66.

20. Henderson WR, Chi EY, Bollinger JG, et al. Importance of group X-secreted phospholipase $A_2$ in allergen-induced airway inflammation and remodeling in a mouse asthma model. J Exp Med 2007;204(4):865–77.

21. Hallstrand TS, Chi EY, Singer AG, et al. Secreted phospholipase $A_2$ group X overexpression in asthma and bronchial hyperresponsiveness. Am J Respir Crit Care Med 2007;176(11):1072–8.

22. Henderson WR, Ye X, Lai Y, et al. Key role of group V secreted phospholipase $A_2$ in Th2 cytokine and dendritic cell-driven airway hyperresponsiveness and remodeling. PLoS One 2013;8(2):e56172.

23. Smith WL, DeWitt DL, Garavito RM. Cyclooxygenases: structural, cellular, and molecular biology. Annu Rev Biochem 2000;69:145–82.

24. Harizi H, Juzan M, Moreau J-F, et al. Prostaglandins inhibit 5-lipoxygenase-activating protein expression and leukotriene $B_4$ production from dendritic cells via an IL-10-dependent mechanism. J Immunol Baltim Md 1950 2003;170(1):139–46.

25. Martel-Pelletier J, Mineau F, Fahmi H, et al. Regulation of the expression of 5-lipoxygenase-activating protein/5-lipoxygenase and the synthesis of leukotriene $B_4$ in osteoarthritic chondrocytes: role of transforming growth factor β and eicosanoids. Arthritis Rheum 2004;50(12):3925–33.

26. Flamand N, Surette ME, Picard S, et al. Cyclic AMP-mediated inhibition of 5-lipoxygenase translocation and leukotriene biosynthesis in human neutrophils. Mol Pharmacol 2002;62(2):250–6.

27. Kay LJ, Yeo WW, Peachell PT. Prostaglandin $E_2$ activates $EP_2$ receptors to inhibit human lung mast cell degranulation. Br J Pharmacol 2006;147(7):707–13.

28. Liu T, Laidlaw TM, Katz HR, et al. Prostaglandin $E_2$ deficiency causes a phenotype of aspirin sensitivity that depends on platelets and cysteinyl leukotrienes. Proc Natl Acad Sci U S A 2013;110(42):16987–92.

29. Säfholm J, Manson ML, Bood J, et al. Prostaglandin $E_2$ inhibits mast cell-dependent bronchoconstriction in human small airways through the E prostanoid subtype 2 receptor. J Allergy Clin Immunol 2015;136(5):1232–9.e1.

30. Corrigan CJ, Napoli RL, Meng Q, et al. Reduced expression of the prostaglandin $E_2$ receptor E-prostanoid 2 on bronchial mucosal leukocytes in patients with aspirin-sensitive asthma. J Allergy Clin Immunol 2012;129(6):1636–46.

31. Pierzchalska M, Szabó Z, Sanak M, et al. Deficient prostaglandin $E_2$ production by bronchial fibroblasts of asthmatic patients, with special reference to aspirin-induced asthma. J Allergy Clin Immunol 2003;111(5):1041–8.

32. Gauvreau GM, Watson RM, O'Byrne PM. Protective effects of inhaled $PGE_2$ on allergen-induced airway responses and airway inflammation. Am J Respir Crit Care Med 1999;159(1):31–6.

33. Sestini P, Armetti L, Gambaro G, et al. Inhaled $PGE_2$ prevents aspirin-induced bronchoconstriction and urinary $LTE_4$ excretion in aspirin-sensitive asthma. Am J Respir Crit Care Med 1996;153(2):572–5.

34. Roca-Ferrer J, Garcia-Garcia FJ, Pereda J, et al. Reduced expression of COXs and production of prostaglandin $E_2$ in patients with nasal polyps with or without aspirin-intolerant asthma. J Allergy Clin Immunol 2011;128(1):66–72.e1.

35. Laidlaw TM, Kidder MS, Bhattacharyya N, et al. Cysteinyl leukotriene overproduction in aspirin-exacerbated respiratory disease is driven by platelet-adherent leukocytes. Blood 2012;119(16):3790–8.

36. Celik G, Bavbek S, Misirligil Z, et al. Release of cysteinyl leukotrienes with aspirin stimulation and the effect of prostaglandin $E_2$ on this release from peripheral blood leucocytes in aspirin-induced asthmatic patients. Clin Exp Allergy 2001; 31(10):1615–22.

37. Ying S, Meng Q, Scadding G, et al. Aspirin-sensitive rhinosinusitis is associated with reduced E-prostanoid 2 receptor expression on nasal mucosal inflammatory cells. J Allergy Clin Immunol 2006;117(2):312–8.

38. Laidlaw TM, Boyce JA. Aspirin-exacerbated respiratory disease-new prime suspects. N Engl J Med 2016;374(5):484–8.

39. Matsuoka T, Hirata M, Tanaka H, et al. Prostaglandin $D_2$ as a mediator of allergic asthma. Science 2000;287(5460):2013–7.

40. Yoshimura T, Yoshikawa M, Otori N, et al. Correlation between the prostaglandin $D_2/E_2$ ratio in nasal polyps and the recalcitrant pathophysiology of chronic rhinosinusitis associated with bronchial asthma. Allergol Int Off J Jpn Soc Allergol 2008;57(4):429–36.

41. Mastalerz L, Celejewska-Wójcik N, Wójcik K, et al. Induced sputum eicosanoids during aspirin bronchial challenge of asthmatic patients with aspirin hypersensitivity. Allergy 2014;69(11):1550–9.

42. Bochenek G, Nagraba K, Nizankowska E, et al. A controlled study of $9\alpha,11\beta$-$PGF_2$ (a prostaglandin $D_2$ metabolite) in plasma and urine of patients with bronchial asthma and healthy controls after aspirin challenge. J Allergy Clin Immunol 2003;111(4):743–9.

43. Mastalerz L, Sanak M, Gawlewicz-Mroczka A, et al. Prostaglandin $E_2$ systemic production in patients with asthma with and without aspirin hypersensitivity. Thorax 2008;63(1):27–34.

44. Daham K, Song W-L, Lawson JA, et al. Effects of celecoxib on major prostaglandins in asthma. Clin Exp Allergy 2011;41(1):36–45.

45. Berges-Gimeno MP, Simon RA, Stevenson DD. Long-term treatment with aspirin desensitization in asthmatic patients with aspirin-exacerbated respiratory disease. J Allergy Clin Immunol 2003;111(1):180–6.

46. Cahill KN, Bensko JC, Boyce JA, et al. Prostaglandin $D_2$: a dominant mediator of aspirin-exacerbated respiratory disease. J Allergy Clin Immunol 2015;135(1):245–52.

47. Maugeri N, Evangelista V, Celardo A, et al. Polymorphonuclear leukocyte-platelet interaction: role of P-selectin in thromboxane $B_2$ and leukotriene $C_4$ cooperative synthesis. Thromb Haemost 1994;72(3):450–6.

48. Christie PE, Tagari P, Ford-Hutchinson AW, et al. Urinary leukotriene $E_4$ concentrations increase after aspirin challenge in aspirin-sensitive asthmatic subjects. Am Rev Respir Dis 1991;143(5 Pt 1):1025–9.

49. Ferreri NR, Howland WC, Stevenson DD, et al. Release of leukotrienes, prostaglandins, and histamine into nasal secretions of aspirin-sensitive asthmatics during reaction to aspirin. Am Rev Respir Dis 1988;137(4):847–54.

50. Hirata H, Arima M, Fukushima Y, et al. Over-expression of the $LTC_4$ synthase gene in mice reproduces human aspirin-induced asthma. Clin Exp Allergy 2011;41(8):1133–42.

51. Buchheit KM, Cahill KN, Katz HR, et al. Thymic stromal lymphopoietin controls prostaglandin $D_2$ generation in patients with aspirin-exacerbated respiratory disease. J Allergy Clin Immunol 2016;137(5):1566–76.e5.

52. Liu T, Kanaoka Y, Barrett NA, et al. Aspirin-exacerbated respiratory disease involves a cysteinyl leukotriene-driven IL-33-mediated mast cell activation pathway. J Immunol Baltim Md 1950 2015;195(8):3537–45.

53. Tager AM, Luster AD. BLT1 and BLT2: the leukotriene $B_4$ receptors. Prostaglandins Leukot Essent Fatty Acids 2003;69(2–3):123–34.

54. Heise CE, O'Dowd BF, Figueroa DJ, et al. Characterization of the human cysteinyl leukotriene 2 receptor. J Biol Chem 2000;275(39):30531–6.

55. Kanaoka Y, Boyce JA. Cysteinyl leukotrienes and their receptors: cellular distribution and function in immune and inflammatory responses. J Immunol Baltim Md 1950 2004;173(3):1503–10.

56. Peters-Golden M, Henderson WR. Leukotrienes. N Engl J Med 2007;357(18):1841–54.

57. Laitinen LA, Laitinen A, Haahtela T, et al. Leukotriene $E_4$ and granulocytic infiltration into asthmatic airways. Lancet Lond Engl 1993;341(8851):989–90.
58. Davidson AB, Lee TH, Scanlon PD, et al. Bronchoconstrictor effects of leukotriene $E_4$ in normal and asthmatic subjects. Am Rev Respir Dis 1987;135(2):333–7.
59. Lee TH, Woszczek G, Farooque SP. Leukotriene $E_4$: perspective on the forgotten mediator. J Allergy Clin Immunol 2009;124(3):417–21.
60. Maekawa A, Kanaoka Y, Xing W, et al. Functional recognition of a distinct receptor preferential for leukotriene $E_4$ in mice lacking the cysteinyl leukotriene 1 and 2 receptors. Proc Natl Acad Sci U S A 2008;105(43):16695–700.
61. Paruchuri S, Tashimo H, Feng C, et al. Leukotriene $E_4$-induced pulmonary inflammation is mediated by the P2Y12 receptor. J Exp Med 2009;206(11):2543–55.
62. Paruchuri S, Jiang Y, Feng C, et al. Leukotriene $E_4$ activates peroxisome proliferator-activated receptor $\gamma$ and induces prostaglandin $D_2$ generation by human mast cells. J Biol Chem 2008;283(24):16477–87.
63. Kanaoka Y, Maekawa A, Austen KF. Identification of GPR99 protein as a potential third cysteinyl leukotriene receptor with a preference for leukotriene $E_4$ ligand. J Biol Chem 2013;288(16):10967–72.
64. Bankova LG, Lai J, Yoshimoto E, et al. Leukotriene $E_4$ elicits respiratory epithelial cell mucin release through the G-protein-coupled receptor, GPR99. Proc Natl Acad Sci U S A 2016;113(22):6242–7.
65. Foster HR, Fuerst E, Branchett W, et al. Leukotriene $E_4$ is a full functional agonist for human cysteinyl leukotriene type 1 receptor-dependent gene expression. Sci Rep 2016;6:20461.
66. Israel E, Fischer AR, Rosenberg MA, et al. The pivotal role of 5-lipoxygenase products in the reaction of aspirin-sensitive asthmatics to aspirin. Am Rev Respir Dis 1993;148(6 Pt 1):1447–51.
67. Pauls JD, Simon RA, Daffern PJ, et al. Lack of effect of the 5-lipoxygenase inhibitor zileuton in blocking oral aspirin challenges in aspirin-sensitive asthmatics. Ann Allergy Asthma Immunol 2000;85(1):40–5.
68. Stevenson DD, Simon RA, Mathison DA, et al. Montelukast is only partially effective in inhibiting aspirin responses in aspirin-sensitive asthmatics. Ann Allergy Asthma Immunol 2000;85(6 Pt 1):477–82.
69. Berges-Gimeno MP, Simon RA, Stevenson DD. The effect of leukotriene-modifier drugs on aspirin-induced asthma and rhinitis reactions. Clin Exp Allergy 2002; 32(10):1491–6.

# Genetic and Epigenetic Components of Aspirin-Exacerbated Respiratory Disease

Amber Dahlin, PhD, MMSc, Scott T. Weiss, MD, MS*

## KEYWORDS

- Cysteinyl leukotriene • Eosinophil • Biomarker • Epigenetics • Polymorphism
- AERD

## KEY POINTS

- Aspirin-exacerbated respiratory disease (AERD) severity and its clinical phenotypes are characterized by genetic variation within pathways for arachidonic acid metabolism, inflammation, and immune responses.
- Epigenetic effects, including DNA methylation and histone protein modification, contribute to regulation of many genes that contribute to inflammatory states in AERD.
- The development of noninvasive, predictive clinical tests using data from genetic, epigenetic, pharmacogenetic, and biomarker studies will improve precision medicine efforts for AERD and asthma treatment.

## INTRODUCTION

Aspirin intolerance is a severe and rare asthmatic endotype, with prevalence rates of 10% in the adult asthmatic population and up to 25% in patients with severe, persistent asthma.[1–4] Consistent with the classification of asthma as a set of individual subtypes of diseases of varying symptoms and severity, AERD is distinguished from other types of severe asthma primarily by its clinical characteristics. The clinical features of AERD include airway obstruction, increased exacerbations, chronic rhinosinusitis, the presence of nasal polyps (NPs), eosinophilia, increased need for systemic glucocorticoids and poor response to asthma controller medication, and an increase in urinary leukotrienes (LTs), both in comparison to aspirin-tolerant asthma (ATA) and after aspirin challenge and symptom exacerbations.[5,6] Due to the discovery

Disclosure Statement: The authors have nothing to disclose. This work was supported by grants from the National Institutes of Health and National Heart, Lung, and Blood Institute (U01HL065899-09 and K12 HL120004-02).
Channing Division of Network Medicine, Brigham and Women's Hospital, Harvard Medical School, 181 Longwood Avenue, Boston, MA 02115, USA
* Corresponding author.
E-mail address: scott.weiss@channing.harvard.edu

Immunol Allergy Clin N Am 36 (2016) 765–789
http://dx.doi.org/10.1016/j.iac.2016.06.010
0889-8561/16/$ – see front matter © 2016 Elsevier Inc. All rights reserved.

that increased production of LTs is a characteristic of AERD, the LT and prostaglandin (PG) production pathways were among the first to be investigated, and the subsequent identification of polymorphisms in LT-related genes in affected patients suggested a pivotal role for genetic variation in the development of AERD.[6–8] As a result, variation in patient genetics has received considerable focus as a potential determinant of AERD pathogenesis.

The observation that severely asthmatic subjects responded favorably to antileukotriene asthma medications contributed further evidence toward a mechanistic role for LTs, while also providing an opportunity for clinicians to more appropriately tailor treatment to a specific patient group.[7,9–12] Subsequent genetic studies revealed considerable evidence for genetic variation in AERD pathophysiology across multiple biological pathways[7,13] as well as variation in interindividual treatment responses to multiple asthma drug classes, including leukotriene modifiers and inhibitors.[14] The exact mechanisms by which LT synthesis becomes dysregulated in AERD, however, are still unknown. Due to corresponding alteration of immune molecules (eg, type 2 helper T cell [$T_H2$] cytokines), PGs (eg, $PGE_2$), and other inflammatory biomarkers (eg, interleukin [IL]-5, periostin, immunoglobulin [Ig] E, apolipoprotein A1, and others), multiple interacting pathways and mechanisms likely also contribute. Evidence that AERD has a heritable basis is minimal, and only two studies reported that 1% to 6% of individuals with AERD had an affected family member.[4,15] The adult onset of AERD, combined with the low genetic penetrance and inconsistent replication of results from genetic associations, point toward involvement of environmental exposures and epigenetic factors in its progression. Achieving a better understanding of the genetic and epigenetic determinants of heterogeneity of AERD through genome-wide and epigenome-wide interrogation is, therefore, anticipated to improve strategies to develop more precisely tailored therapeutic agents, treatment regimens, and potentially cures for the disease.

## UPDATE ON THE GENETICS OF ASPIRIN-EXACERBATED RESPIRATORY DISEASE

The quest to discover determinants of AERD (and its unique clinical features) has yielded a rapidly increasing number of candidate gene and genetic association studies. These studies reveal mechanistic insights into the molecular pathways for aspirin hypersensitivity, including arachidonic acid metabolism and cysteinyl leukotriene (CysLT) production, inflammatory cascades initiated by eosinophils, mast cells, platelets, airway epithelial cells, and others. For reference, this article summarizes the major results from these studies in **Table 1**. Findings from many of these studies are conflicting, however, and a majority of reported associations lack replication. This section provides a comprehensive update of the status of genetic investigations of aspirin-sensitive asthma and AERD, highlighting major discoveries published within the past several years. In addition to discussing genetics association studies of AERD risk, recent findings are presented from investigations of genetic markers associated with two predominant AERD clinical features—nasal polyposis[2] and eosiniophilia.[6]

### Genetic Markers Associated with Disease Status and Clinical Features of Aspirin-Exacerbated Respiratory Disease

#### Aspirin-exacerbated respiratory disease susceptibility
Previous studies have yielded a substantial number of genes and genetic markers associated with AERD affection status and/or clinical phenotypes (summarized in **Table 1**). This section discusses recent discoveries with compelling evidence for a role in AERD pathogenesis.

**Table 1**
Summary of results from genetic studies of aspirin-sensitive asthma

| Pathway | Gene Symbol | Polymorphism(s) | Major Association(s), Clinical Phenotype(s), or Functional Effect(s) | Study Population(s) and Ethnicities[a] | Replication Population(s) and Ethnicities[a] | Study Type | References (PMID) |
|---|---|---|---|---|---|---|---|
| Airway cell function and response | ADRB2 | rs1042713 | Reference homozygous genotype is more common in ATA vs AERD; no effects on lung function measures or IgE | 95 AERD; 300 ATA; 100 NC; Asian (Japanese) | | CGAS | 21829036 |
| | EMID2 | EMID2_BL2_ht2 | Differences in $\Delta FEV_1$ by aspirin provocation in AIA vs ATA | 163 AIA; 429 ATA; Asian (Korean) | | CGAS | 21086123 |
| | KIF3A | rs3756775 | Associated with the rate of $FEV_1$ decline by aspirin provocation in AIA | 103 AIA; 268 ATA; Asian (Korean) | | CGAS | 20922562 |
| | SPINK5 | G1258A, A1103G | Heterozygous genotypes were more frequently observed in AIA | 15 CRSsNP; 59 CRSwNP (18 AIA); 30 NC; white (European) | | CGAS | 22570283 |

(continued on next page)

**Table 1**
*(continued)*

| Pathway | Gene Symbol | Polymorphism(s) | Major Association(s), Clinical Phenotype(s), or Functional Effect(s) | Study Population(s) and Ethnicities[a] | Replication Population(s) and Ethnicities[a] | Study Type | References (PMID) |
|---|---|---|---|---|---|---|---|
| Arachidonic acid metabolism and signaling | LTC4S | −444A > C | Association with ATA but not AIA | 356 AIA; 840 ATA; 902 NC; Multiple (white, Asian, African American) | | MA | 22884858 |
| | ALOX5 | ht1[GCGA] | Increased frequency of haplotype for AIA | 93 AIA; 181 ATA; 123 NC; Asian (Korean) | | CGAS | 14749922 |
| | COX2 | −765G > C | CC homozygosity was associated with disease severity; increased PG production by monocytes | 112 AIA; 198 ATA; 547 NC; white (Polish) | | CGAS | 15316498 |
| | CYP2C19 | rs4244285, rs4986893 | Lower % predicted $FEV_1$ after aspirin provocation in AERD | 100 AERD; 300 ATA; 100 NC; Asian (Japanese) | | CGAS | 21855977 |
| | CYSLTR1 | −634C > T, −475A > C, −336A > G | Higher frequency and promoter activity of ht(TCG) in AERD | 105 AIA; 110 ATA; 125 NC; Asian (Korean) | | CGAS | 16630147 |
| | CYSLTR2 | −819T > G, 2078C > T, 2534A > G | Increased frequency of minor alleles and decline in $FEV_1$ by aspirin provocation in AIA | 86 AIA; 134 ATA; 152 NC; Asian (Korean) | | CGAS | 15970796 |
| | EP2 | uS5, uS5b, uS7 | Associated with AIA; reduced transcriptional activity of the EP2 gene | 87 AIA; 192 ATA; 96 NC; Asian (Japanese) | 198 AIA; 282 ATA; 274 NC; Asian (Japanese) | CGAS | 15496426 |
| | NAT2 | −9246G > C | Associated with risk of AIA | 170 AIA; 268 ATA; Asian (Korean) | | CGAS | 20602614 |
| | PTGDR | −613C > T, −549T > C, −441C > T, −197T > C | Diplotype is more frequent in patients with aspirin triad, asthma and aspirin intolerance than NC | 145 Asthma + NP; 81 AIA + NP; 75 aspirin triad + NP; 245 NC; white (Spanish) | | CGAS | 23101307 |
| | PTGER | rs7543182, rs959 | Associated with risk of AIA in the discovery population | 137 AIA; 268 ATA; Asian (Korean) | 106 AIA; 651 ATA; Asian (Korean) | CGAS | 20587336 |

| | Gene | Variant | Description | Sample | | PMID |
|---|---|---|---|---|---|---|
| | TBXA2R | rs11085026 | Increased association and greater percent fall of $FEV_1$ after aspirin provocation for AIA | 93 AIA; 172 ATA; 118 NC; Asian (Korean) | CGAS | 15898979 |
| | TBXAS1 | rs6962291 | Lower frequency of minor allele; association with fall of $FEV_1$ after aspirin provocation for AIA | 200 AIA; 270 ATA; Asian (Korean) | CGAS | 21449675 |
| Inflammatory responses | ACE | −262A > T, −115T > C | Increased risk of AIA; homozygotes for minor alleles had a greater decline in $FEV_1$ after aspirin provocation than reference homozygotes | 81 AIA; 231 ATA; 181 NC; Asian (Korean) | CGAS | 18727619 |
| | AGT | p2401C > G, p2476C > T | Increased MAF in AIA cases resistant to montelukast treatment; associated with modified response to montelukast | 56 AIA; Asian (Korean) | CGAS | 21624492 |
| | CACNG6 | rs192808; CACNG6_BL1_ht6 | Associated with increased risk of AIA | 102 AIA; 429 ATA; Asian (Korean) | CGAS | 20860846 |
| | CCR3 | −520T > C | Predictive accuracy for AIA >65% (with B2ADR 46A > G, CysLTR1−634C > T, and FCER1B−109T > C) | 94 AIA; 152 ATA; Asian (Korean) | CGAS | 18379861 |
| | CRTH2 | −446T > C | Serum eotaxin-2 was significantly higher in AERD with the TT genotype than CT/CC | 107 AERD; 115 ATA; 133 NC; Asian (Korean) | CGAS | 19796209 |
| | ECP | | mRNA and protein expression increased in AERD | 15 AERD; 15 CRSwNP; unspecified (United States) | EP | 26067893 |
| | ERAS | | mRNA expression was increased in AIA vs controls | 11 AIA; 7 ATA; 15 NC; white (Polish) | EP | 26646719 |
| | FOSL1 | | mRNA and protein expression reduced in AIA vs controls | 11 AIA; 7 ATA; 15 NC; white (Polish) | EP | 26646719 |

(continued on next page)

**Table 1**
*(continued)*

| Pathway | Gene Symbol | Polymorphism(s) | Major Association(s), Clinical Phenotype(s), or Functional Effect(s) | Study Population(s) and Ethnicities[a] | Replication Population(s) and Ethnicities[a] | Study Type | References (PMID) |
|---|---|---|---|---|---|---|---|
| | HSPA1B | rs6457452, rs1061581 | Increased MAF in AERD vs ATA; variance in eosinophil count by SNP for AERD vs ATA | 102 AERD; 300 ATA; 100 NC; Asian (Japanese) | | CGAS | 23392055 |
| | IL13 | rs1800925 | Higher MAF in AERD vs ATA | 95 AERD; 300 ATA; 100 NC; Asian (Japanese) | | CGAS | 22123380 |
| | | −1510A > C | Reduced MAF in AIA vs ATA for AA genotype vs CC genotype of −1510A > C | 162 AIA; 301 ATA; 430 NC; Asian (Japanese) | | | 20358028 |
| | NOS2A | [(CCTTT)n] | Association of more than 14 repeats of the NOS2A (CCTTT) repeat cluster in AIA and aspirin triad than NC | 81 AIA; 75 aspirin triad; 245 NC; white (Spanish) | | CGAS | 23101307 |
| | PPARG | 82466C > T | Increased MAF in AIA vs ATA | 60 AIA; 343 ATA; 449 NC; Asian (Korean) | | CGAS | 20224667 |
| | RAB1A | 14,444T > G, 41,170C > G | Increased MAF in AIA vs ATA, and association with $FEV_1$ decline after aspirin provocation | 181 AIA; 1016 ATA; Asian (Korean) | | CGAS | 24555545 |
| | SLC6A12 | rs557881 | Associated with AIA and decline in $FEV_1$ after aspirin provocation | 163 AIA; 429 ATA; Asian (Korean) | | CGAS | 20597903 |
| | STK10 | rs2306961 | Associated with AIA | 163 AIA; 429 ATA; Asian (Korean) | | CGAS | 21905501 |

| Category | Gene | Variant | Description | Population | Population 2 | Study | PMID |
|---|---|---|---|---|---|---|---|
| Initiation of immune responses | CIITA | rs1139564 | Associated with nasal polyposis in AERD | 158 AERD; 309 ATA; Asian (Korean) | | CGAS | 23292525 |
| | CNPY3 | | mRNA expression reduced in AIA vs controls | 11 AIA; 7 ATA; 15 NC; white (Polish) | | EP | 26646719 |
| | GM-CSF | | Elevated mRNA and protein in AERD | 15 AERD; 15 CRSwNP; (United States) | | EP | 26067893 |
| | HLADPB1 | rs3128965 | Increased MAF, bronchial hyperresponsiveness to inhaled aspirin and methacholine, and higher 15-HETE levels | 179 AERD; 1989 HC; Asian (Korean) | 264 AERD; 387 ATA; 238 NC; Asian (Korean) | GWAS | 25536158 |
| | | rs1042151 | Increased AERD susceptibility and gene dose effect for percent decline in FEV$_1$ after aspirin provocation | 117 AERD; 685 ATA; Asian (Korean) | 142 AERD; 946 ATA; Asian (Korean) | GWAS | 23180272 |
| | | exm537513 | Increased risk of AERD; predictive for AERD susceptibility vs ATA | 165 AERD; 397 ATA; 398 NC; Asian (Korean) | | EWAS | 25372592 |
| | | DPB1*0301 | Increased MAF in AIA | 59 AIA; 57 ATA; 48 NC; white (Polish) | | CGAS | 9179433 |
| | HLADPB2 | exm-rs3129294 | Predictive for AERD susceptibility vs ATA | 165 AERD; 397 ATA; 398 NC; Asian (Korean) | | EWAS | 25372592 |
| | HLADQA1 | DQA1*0301, DQA1*0201, DQA1*0501 | Haplotypes associated with AERD risk | 33 AERD; 17 ATA; 100 NC | | CGAS | 25975240 |
| | HLADQB1 | DQB1*0301 | Lower MAF for AERD vs ATA | 33 AERD; 17 ATA; 100 NC | | CGAS | 25975240 |
| | | DQB1*0302 | Lower MAF in poor responders to aspirin desensitization | 16 AERD | | CGAS | 26366802 |
| | HLADRB1 | DRB1*04, DRB1*07, DRB1*011 | Haplotypes associated with AERD risk | 33 AERD; 17 ATA; 100 NC | | CGAS | 25975240 |
| | HLADRB3 | | MAF lower for AERD vs ATA | 33 AERD; 17 ATA; 100 NC | | CGAS | 25975240 |
| | HLADRB4 | | MAF higher for AERD vs ATA | 33 AERD; 17 ATA; 100 NC | | CGAS | 25975240 |
| | IL10/TGFb | −1082A > G, −509C > T | −1082A/G associated with AIA; synergistic effect between TGF-β1 −509C/T and IL-10 −1082A/G in AIA | 173 AIA; 260 ATA; 448 NC; Asian (Korean) | | CGAS | 19222424 |

(continued on next page)

**Table 1**
*(continued)*

| Pathway | Gene Symbol | Polymorphism(s) | Major Association(s), Clinical Phenotype(s), or Functional Effect(s) | Study Population(s) and Ethnicities[a] | Replication Population(s) and Ethnicities[a] | Study Type | References (PMID) |
|---|---|---|---|---|---|---|---|
| | IL17RA | −1075A > G, −947A > G, −50C > T, BL1_ht1 | MAF lower for AERD vs ATA | 143 AERD; 411 ATA; 825 NC; Asian (Korean) | | CGAS | 23220496 |
| | IL4 | −589T > C, −33C | Both associated with AIA risk; MAF for −589T > C was higher in the AIA vs ATA and associated with a gene dose-dependent decline in FEV$_1$ after aspirin provocation | 103 AIA; 270 ATA; Asian (Korean) | | CGAS | 20921925 |
| | IL5RA | −5993G > A | AA genotype had increased IgE responses to staphylococcal enterotoxin A in AERD patients | 139 AERD; 171 ATA; 160 NC; Asian (Korean) | | CGAS | 23470716 |
| | MCP-1 | | Elevated mRNA and protein in AERD | 15 AERD; 15 CRSwNP; unspecified (United States) | | EP | 26067893 |
| | TAP2 | Multiple haplotypes | Associated with FEV$_1$ decline by aspirin provocation in AERD | 93 AERD; 96 ATA; Asian (Korean) | | CGAS | 21796142 |
| | TLR3 | −299698G > T, 293391G > A | Increased MAF in AERD vs ATA for −29969G > A'; reduced MAF 2200698G > T in AERD vs ATA | 203 AERD; 254 ATA; 274 NC; Asian (Korean) | | CGAS | 21461252 |
| | UBE3C | rs3802122, rs6979947 rs10949635 | Lower risk for AIA | 163 AIA; 429 ATA; Asian (Korean) | | CGAS | 20934631 |
| | | | Associated with nasal polyposis in ATA vs AERD | 114 AERD; 353 ATA; Asian (Korean) | | CGAS | 21881582 |
| Asthma/ NSAID response | CEP68 | CEP68_ht4 (T-G-A-A-A-C-G), rs7572857 | Associated with increased risk of AIA and higher decline of FEV$_1$ after aspirin provocation | 80 AIA; 100 ATA; Asian (Korean) | 163 AIA; 429 ATA; Asian (Korean) | GWAS | 21072201 |
| | DPP10 | rs17048175 | Association with AERD but not ATA | 274 AERD; 272 ATA; 99 NC; Asian (Korean) | | CGAS | 25592153 |

*Abbreviations:* A/G, A to G transition; C/T, C to T transition; CGAS, candidate gene association study; CRSsNP, chronic rhinosinusitis without nasal polyposis; CRSwNP, chronic rhinosinusitis with nasal polyposis; EP, expression profiling; EWAS, exome-wide association study; ht(TCG), haplotype TCG; MA, meta-analysis; NC, normal (non-asthmatic) controls; PMID, PubMed unique identifier; TGF, transforming growth factor.

[a] Discovery/replication population and their race/ethnicity (if specified)

The best mechanistic evidence for AERD pathogenesis supports intrinsic dysregulation of the activity of the 5-lipoxygenase (LO)/LTC$_4$S pathway, leading to increased recruitment and tissue infiltration of immune effectors. These effects are mediated largely by alterations in genes that are directly involved in arachidonic acid metabolism and signaling, namely LTC4S,[16,17] ALOX5,[18,19] CYSLTR1,[20–22] CYSLTR2,[20,21] TBX21,[23] EP2,[24] and COX2.[25,26] A summary of the clinical evidence for these associations is presented in **Table 1**. The arachidonic acid metabolism signaling pathway genes LTC4S, ALOX5, CYSLTR1, and CYSLTR2 represent the most important candidate genes in this pathway and have the strongest evidence for a role in AERD pathogenesis. An LTC4S−444A/C promoter single nucleotide polymorphism (SNP) (rs730012) is among the most widely reported variants associated with AERD, although its association with AERD across studies is inconsistent.[27–31] A recent meta-analysis of 13 case-control studies of asthma revealed significant increased risk in ATA populations carrying the CC or AC genotype versus AA genotype (odds ratio [OR] 1.36; 95% CI, 1.12–1.65; P = .002) but not in aspirin-intolerant groups (OR 1.16; 95% CI, 0.89–1.52; P = .27).[31] Therefore, variation in LTC4S, although consistently associated with ATA, may not be consistently related to AERD across populations. Three ALOX5 promoter variants have been associated with AERD and/or its severity of hyper-responsiveness[19,32,33] (see **Table 1**). New ALOX5 variants associated with AERD, however, have not been identified. The CYSLTR1 and CYSLTR2 leukotriene receptor genes are among the most important for leukotriene signaling and are pharmacologic targets for montelukast, the gold standard prescribed medication for AERD symptom control.[34–36] CYSLTR1 is overexpressed in nasal tissues of AERD patients, and 3 promoter SNPs in CYSLTR1 have been associated with both AERD status and higher CYSLTR1 promoter activity, suggesting that functional variation driving overexpression of this receptor underlies its pathologic roles in LT signaling in AERD[37,38] (see **Table 1**). Polymorphisms in CYSLTR2 are also associated with AERD and forced expiratory volume in the first second of expiration (FEV$_1$) decline after aspirin provocation test (see **Table 1**), suggesting a role for this receptor as well in driving clinical features of AERD.

In addition to these genes, novel candidate genes within the arachidonic acid pathway were recently evaluated for their association with AERD. Prior genetic studies demonstrated an association of asthma susceptibility with dipeptidyl-peptidase 10 (DPP10), which encodes a potentially nonfunctional serine protease with unknown biological roles.[39,40] The association was also correlated with serum DPP10 levels. This association, and correlation with serum DPP10, was replicated in a follow-up association study in 272 AERD patients, 272 ATA patients, and 99 healthy controls of Korean ethnicity.[41] In addition, there was a significant correlation of serum DPP10 levels with the serum levels of 15-hydroxyeicosatetraenoic acid (HETE), an arachidonic acid pathway metabolite that is released at higher levels in eosinophils from severely affected AERD patients.[41] Although the biological roles of DPP10 in asthma tolerant asthma are unclear, its increased serum protein levels and correlation with serum 15-HETE suggest that these may be protein biomarkers for AERD.[41] Another arachidonic acid pathway gene, FABP1, was suspected of involvement in AERD due to its roles in regulating bioactive lipid mediators; however, no significant association between the FABP1 polymorphisms and AERD or lung function was found.[42] There is reasonably strong evidence implicating LTs and DPP10 in AERD pathogenesis. What remains unclear is what role genetic susceptibility plays in disease onset and whether other pathways are involved in disease pathogenesis.

### Genetic associations with nasal polyposis in aspirin-exacerbated respiratory disease/aspirin-induced asthma

AERD comprises up to 30% of asthmatics with NPs.[25,43] Inflammatory mediators in the $T_H2$ cytokine pathway may drive the development of symptoms characteristic of AERD, including chronic rhinosinusitis associated with nasal polyposis.[43–45] Patients with AERD undergo a greater frequency of revision sinonasal surgeries and have a higher rate of postsurgical symptomatic recurrence than patients with non–AERD-related chronic rhinosinusitis with NPs.[44–46] The genetic and molecular mechanisms, however, that can differentiate this particular AERD phenotype from non-AERD phenotypes with nasal polyposis are unclear. Comparison of an inflammatory response signature, including $T_H2$ and non-$T_H2$ cytokine and chemokine–encoding genes, identified from microarray expression profiling of inflammatory mediators within NP samples from patients with chronic rhinosinusitis versus patients with AERD, revealed significantly elevated expression of 5 mediators (eosinophilic cationic protein [ECP], GM-CSF, SDF-1α and SDF1β, MCP-1, and IL10) and reduced expression of tissue plasminogen activator in the NPs of AERD.[47] AERD NPs also contained significantly elevated protein levels of ECP, GM-CSF and MCP-1 compared with the chronic rhinosinusitis samples,[47] as well as increased eosinophilia. No corresponding increase in $T_H2$-specific protein expression was associated, however, with eosinophil proliferation and recruitment in AERD samples, suggesting that other non-$T_H2$ processes, may be important for AERD pathogenesis.[47]

A major histocompatibility complex (MHC)-related gene, class II MHC transactivator (CIITA), is expressed in NPs, and polymorphisms in this gene are associated with the development of multiple immune-related disorders due to the importance of MHC genes in regulating immune responses.[48] Eighteen CIITA SNPs hypothesized to play a role in AERD were genotyped in 158 AERD patients and 309 ATA patients of Korean ancestry, and one SNP, rs1139564, was nominally associated with NPs in the AERD group.[48] This association did not persist, however, after multiple test corrections.[48]

Because eicosanoids and their receptors are up-regulated in inflammatory cells within NP tissue,[49,50] corresponding to high levels of LTC4S,[51] CYSLTR1,[20] and PTGDR,[25] transcript expression in NPs, altered leukotriene metabolism is also implicated in the development of this phenotype in AERD. A candidate gene study of variants in LTC4S (−444A > C), PTGDR (−613C > T, −549T > C, −441C > T, and −197T > C), CYSLTR1 (927T > C), and NOS2A [(CCTTT)n] in samples from 81 asthmatics with nasal polyposis and aspirin intolerance, 75 patients with nasal polyposis and the aspirin triad, and 245 unaffected controls, revealed a significant association for more than 14 repeats of the NOS2A (CCTTT) repeat cluster in patients with aspirin intolerance (OR 3.68; 95% CI, 1.31–10.36; $P$ = .009) and in patients with the aspirin triad (OR 0.25; 95% CI, 0.09–0.72; $P$ = .005).[52] In addition, the PTGDR diplotype CCCT/CCCC (−613CC, −549CC, −441CC, and −197TC) occurred more frequently among patients with the aspirin triad (OR 3.16; 95% CI, 1.05–9.49; $P$ = .04).[52] Nitric oxide is an important inflammatory mediator produced at high levels during inflammatory states that is carried out predominantly by NOS2A in the paranasal sinuses.[53] Modification of NOS2A transcript expression may be crucial for development of NPs,[54] pointing toward an important role for this gene in development of this phenotype.

In summary, genetic studies of nasal polyposis in AERD/aspirin-induced asthma (AIA) implicate inflammation and the eicosanoid pathway.

### Genetic associations with eosinophilia in aspirin-exacerbated respiratory disease/aspirin-induced asthma

Persistent eosinophilia and cytokine overproduction are critical clinical features of AERD[47]; furthermore, eosinophil activation and migration require the presence of cytokines and other immune mediators. Eosinophilia is a $T_H2$ cytokine–dependent process, and expression of IL-4, IL-5, IL-13, and other cytokines correlates with eosinophilic infiltration.[43,47] $T_H2$ cytokine IL-5 receptor alpha (*IL5RA*) polymorphisms have been reported in asthma and allergic diseases and are associated with increased levels of peripheral blood eosinophils, although a direct association with AERD has not been clarified. In a recent study to determine whether *IL5RA* polymorphisms were involved in eosinophil activation in AERD, 139 AERD patients, 171 ATA patients, and 160 normal controls of Korean ancestry were genotyped for 3 suspected *IL5RA* SNPs (−5993G > A, −5567C > G, and −5091G > A) and a case-control analysis and functional characterization of the SNPs were performed.[55] AERD patients with *IL5RA* −5993AA demonstrated a higher IgE to staphylococcal enterotoxin A ratio than heterozygotes or those possessing the reference allele.[55] Furthermore, −5993A demonstrated altered promoter activity by luciferase reporter assay and differential binding of nuclear extracts by EMSA.[55] The investigators conclude that *IL5RA* −5993G > A may, therefore, contribute to eosinophil responses in AERD patients.[55]

In addition to IL5, evidence exists for the recently described IL-17 cytokine family in inflammatory cell recruitment and allergic response.[56,57] Polymorphisms in the IL-17A receptor gene, *IL17RA*, are associated with asthma, and IL-17A activation induces activation of signaling molecules, such as nuclear factor (NF)-κB, that regulate inflammatory processes in human airway cells.[58] In a recent candidate gene study in a Korean population, 15 SNPs in *IL17RA* were analyzed and functionally characterized in 143 patients with AERD, 411 patients with ATA, and 825 normal controls.[59] Three *IL17RA* SNPs (−1075A > G, −947A > G, and −50C > T) were significantly associated with the risk of aspirin intolerance as well as the rate of decline in FEV $_1$ after aspirin challenge, although the minor allele frequencies (MAFs) for all 3 SNPs were significantly lower for AERD.[59] Finally, *IL17RA* expression in CD14$^+$ monocytes from asthmatic patients with all 3 minor allele genotypes for *IL17RA* −1075A > G, −947A > G, and −50C > T was significantly higher than for the reference homozygotes.[59] The minor alleles of the 3 SNPs may, therefore, have protective effects for AERD, presumably by limiting *IL17RA* expression.[59]

The MHC II HLA locus is involved in T-cell activation and has been shown in multiple genetic investigations to have strong associations with asthma. To date, the best genetic marker for AERD is *HLADPB1*0301*, which is also associated with a higher leukotriene receptor antagonist dose to control symptoms and a higher prevalence of chronic rhinosinusitis.[60–62] A recent genetic association study of *HLA-DRB, HLA-DQA1,* and *HLA-DQB1* genotypes in 33 patients with AERD, 17 patients with ATA, and 100 healthy controls was performed after an oral aspirin challenge.[63] In comparison to the controls, frequencies of *HLA-DQB1*0302* and *HLA-DRB1*04* and the haplotypes *HLA-DRB1*04/DQA1*0301/DQB1*0302* and *HLA-DRB1*07/DQA1*0201/DQB1*0201* were higher in patients with AERD whereas *HLA-DQB1*0301, HLA-DQA1*0501, HLA-DRB1*11,* and *HLA-DRB3* allele frequencies were significantly lower.[63] Furthermore, in contrast to ATA patients, patients with AERD had lower frequencies of *HLA-DQB1*0301* and *HLA-DRB1*011.*[63]

The infiltration of eosinophils characteristic of AERD is also promoted by their release of CysLTs. In contrast to ATA with eosinophilic sinusitis, AERD patients show increased expression of leukotriene receptors and hyper-reactivity to CysLTs.[43] Distinguishing the characteristics of eosinophilia occurring in AERD from eosinophilia occurring in ATA may shed light on unique cellular and molecular features of the disorders, facilitating greater understanding of these endotypes, and thus provide opportunities for more precise treatment. Steinke and colleagues[64] profiled the expression of type 1 helper T cell ($T_H1$) and $T_H2$ cytokines in tissue samples from 30 asthmatics with chronic hyperplastic eosinophilic sinusitis, 15 patients with AERD, and 9 healthy controls, using quantitative real-time polymerase chain reaiton.[64] The investigators determined that although a $T_H2$ cytokine signature, as shown by increased expression of IL-4, IL-5, and IL-13, compared with control tissue dominated in both AERD and ATA, AERD alone demonstrated overexpression of $T_H1$ cytokine interferon (IFN)-$\gamma$, which was also determined as originating from eosinophils through flow cytometry and histologic studies.[64] Furthermore, in addition to priming these eosinophils, IFN-$\gamma$ increased the expression of genes involved in leukotriene biosynthesis and CysLT secretion.[64] IFN-$\gamma$ increases CysLT receptor expression on circulating eosinophils and also increased *LTC4S, CYSLT1*, and *CYSLT2* mRNA expression in both mature eosinophils as well as their progenitors, coincident with a significantly enhanced capability of eosinophils to degranulate and secrete CysLTs after stimulation with IFN-$\gamma$.[64,65] These findings suggest that IFN-$\gamma$ may uniquely drive the CysLT overproduction in AERD and may represent an important diagnostic marker.

Additional genes that may regulate proinflammatory cellular responses, including the Ras oncogenes and heat shock proteins (HSPs), have also been recently investigated. *RAB1A* encodes a Ras family GTPase that may contribute to eosinophilia and immune responses in AERD by regulating vesicle exocytosis in activated immune cells. Eight polymorphisms in the *RAB1A* gene were analyzed for associations with the risk of AERD in 181 asthmatic subjects with aspirin intolerance and 1016 non–aspirin-intolerant asthmatic controls.[66] Two SNPs, *RAB1A* 14444G > T and *RAB1A* 41170C > G, were associated with aspirin hypersensitivity and the MAFs of these SNPs were also higher in this group.[66] In addition, the *RAB1A* 14444TT and *RAB1A* 41170GG carriers showed a greater decline in FEV$_1$ after oral aspirin challenge, with heterozygotes for both SNPs demonstrating intermediate levels of FEV$_1$ decline.[66] The Ras family GTPases regulate production of inflammatory mediators,[67] and granule release from platelets, eosinophils, and neutrophils requires RAB1A activation.[68] These data suggest that *RAB1A*, and potentially other members of the Ras oncogene family, may therefore contribute to the development of AERD and merit further investigation.

The HSP family members, in particular HSP70, are correlated with asthma severity and eosinophilia and overexpressed in the asthmatic airway.[69,70] The role of HSPs in allergic asthma, however, is unclear. To investigate the hypothesis that HSP70 variation contributes to AERD susceptibility, a recent study evaluated the association of 2 candidate HSP70 polymorphisms—*HSPA1B*-179C > T and *HSPA1B*-1267A > G (rs6457452 and rs1061581)—in 102 asthmatics with AERD, 300 asthmatics with ATA, and 100 normal healthy controls, all of Japanese descent.[71] In patients with AERD, compared with the ATA group, frequency of the *HSPA1B*-179CT/TT genotype was higher than that of the CC genotype, and the GG genotype of the *HSPA1B*-1267GG was also higher than that of the GA/AA genotype; furthermore, frequency of the *HSPA1B*-179C/1267A haplotype was also higher in the AERD group versus the ATA group and was associated with a significantly increased risk of AERD (OR 3.154; 95% CI, 1.916–5.193).[71] Finally, AERD patients demonstrated a significant variation in eosinophil count by *HSP* SNP genotype, whereas the aspirin-tolerant group did not.[71] Although the molecular mechanisms of HSP70 variation and eosinophilia in AERD were not investigated in this study, the investigators suggest that, as a possible mechanism, because the HSP-encoding genes are located within the MHC III region,[72] the HSP70 SNPs may be in linkage with other SNPs within this region, which is also adjacent to *TNF*, and that could functionally contribute to this association.[71]

*Genome-wide Approaches for Investigating Genetic Relationships in Aspirin-Exacerbated Respiratory Disease*

To date, multiple genetic risk factors for AERD have been identified through candidate gene studies and genome-wide association studies (GWAS) (see **Table 1**). The latest GWAS of AERD, conducted in 2014, analyzed 2379 subjects and also replicated initial findings in an independent cohort of 264 AERD patients, 238 healthy controls, and 387 patients with ATA.[73] Using the Affymetrix Genome-Wide Human SNP Array, Kim and colleagues[73] profiled 275,862 SNPs from 179 AERD patients, 211 patients with aspirin-exacerbated cutaneous disease (AECD), and 1989 healthy control subjects. Although none of the SNP associations achieved genome-wide significance, rs3128965 in *HLA-DPB1* approached genome-wide significance and was associated with AERD in both the discovery and replication populations.[73] Furthermore, asthmatic patients carrying the minor allele of this SNP demonstrated significantly enhanced bronchial hyper-responsiveness to aspirin and methacholine, in addition to higher 15-HETE levels.[73] These data suggest that rs3128965 could represent a potential diagnostic genetic marker for AERD. A prior GWAS had also identified a SNP in *HLA-DPB1* (rs1042151) associated with AERD.[74] In this study, 430,486 SNPs were analyzed for association with AERD, using the Human660W BeadChip (Illumina), in 117 subjects with AERD and 685 ATA patients.[74] None of the SNPs achieved genome-wide significance; however, rs2281389 near *HLA-DPB1* was most strongly associated with AERD (OR 2.41; $P = 5.69 \times 10\text{–}6$).[74] The top 49 SNPs associated with AERD risk were also associated with significant decline of $FEV_1$ after aspirin challenge.[74] For replication, 702 SNPs in the 14 genes were genotyped in 142 AERD and 996 ATA subjects, and a nonsynonymous SNP in *HLA-DPB1*, rs1042151, showed the highest association with the risk of AERD.[74] For reference, the results of earlier GWAS of AERD and AIA are provided in **Table 1**.

Although candidate gene studies have yielded a wealth of information on AERD genotype-phenotype associations, these hypothesis-driven approaches necessarily focus on a small number of genes and, therefore, exclude loci that could also have direct functional importance for the phenotype. Comparing gene expression and whole-sequence profiles from AERD cases and non-AERD asthmatics or healthy controls using whole-genome microarray expression profiling and next-generation sequencing methods provides a discovery-based approach to interrogate mRNA transcripts across the genome with specific correlation to the phenotype. A combined approach using microarray expression profiling and a candidate gene analysis in peripheral blood mononuclear cells (PBMCs) from a small white population identified 3 genes with expression profiles that significantly differed between AIA versus ATA and/or AIA versus healthy subjects.[75] In particular, expression of *CNPY3* and *FOSL1* was significantly lower in AIA versus healthy controls, whereas *ERAS* expression was increased. Protein expression of *FOSL1* in PBMCs was also significantly lower for AIA than the control groups.[75] Although the study lacked mechanistic investigation of these novel candidate genes for AERD, the investigators suggest these genes could participate in innate immune response pathways and pathways for tissue/cell remodeling and airway hyper-responsiveness that contribute to the pathogenesis of AERD.[75]

Genomic studies of complex diseases are increasingly focusing on elucidating the impact of coding variants, which are more likely to be rare and to have larger effect sizes corresponding to their functional significance for gene expression. Shin and colleagues[76] recently used an exome-wide profiling approach using the HumanExome BeadChip v1.1 (Illumina) to identify novel, rare, and exonic SNPs associated with

AERD status in 165 AERD patients, 397 patients with ATA, and 398 normal controls of Korean ancestry. After filtering and quality control of genotype data, more than 54,000 SNPs remained and were evaluated for association with AERD risk.[76] A SNP in HLA-DPB1, exm537513, achieved genome-wide significance and was associated with increased risk of AERD (OR 3.28; P value of $3.4 \times 10^{-8}$).[76] From the top 100 SNP associations, the P values of remaining top 10 SNPs ranged from $3.4 \times 10^{-8}$ to $2.4 \times 10^{-4}$ with ORs from 0.13 to 13.61.[76] Three additional exonic SNPs on HLA-DPB1 (exm537513, exm537522, and exm537523) were also present among the top 20 SNPs. A prior GWAS[77] had identified exm537522 (also annotated as rs1042151 in that study) as having the strongest association with AERD susceptibility; therefore, the investigators replicated one of their top associations from a previous study.[76] To develop a predictive model for AERD risk, the investigators selected the best combination of the top 10 SNPs that could discriminate between AERD and ATA, using multiple logistic regression, and calculated receiver operating characteristic (ROC) curves and area under the curve (AUC) values for each combination model.[76] A combination model of 7 SNPs (exm537513, exm83523, exm1884673, exm538564, exm2264237, exm396794, and exm791954) in HLA-DPB1, HLA-DPA1, and HLA-DPB2 could predict AERD versus non-AERD status (AUC of 0.75; 34% sensitivity and 93% specificity).[76] A major limitation of this study is that no replication was performed. In summary, GWAS tend to support the involvement of the HLA locus in the pathogenesis of AERD.

### Limitations of These Studies

A significant limitation of genetic studies of AERD is that few have replicated their associations. Moreover, a majority of the top associations lacked genome-wide or experiment-wide significance. Furthermore, the lack of uniformity in genetic associations across diverse populations confounds generalizability of these loci to the AERD patient population. A consistent limitation of these, and clinical genetic studies in general, is the limited numbers of patients available for study, which greatly limits statistical power to detect actual SNP associations with phenotype. Genome-wide association studies also typically exclude rare variants (MAF <1%) that are more likely to be present in coding regions and have more direct correlations with function, limiting the ability to detect functional associations. Finally, a majority of studies also lack experimental validation of their genetic findings, limiting the ability to discern the molecular function of these variations and their potential clinical consequences. Future genetic studies of AERD must consider replication of initial findings across well-powered populations and include functional validation in appropriate cellular models.

## EPIGENETICS OF ASPIRIN-EXACERBATED RESPIRATORY DISEASE

Epigenetic modifications include methylation of CpG islands in gene promoter regions, and the acetylation and deacetylation of histone proteins, all of which can significantly alter chromatin unfolding and hence gene expression. Furthermore, epigenetic modification patterns can vary greatly across cell and tissue types. There is a correlation between the rise in asthma susceptibility and early exposure to environmental allergens during development, which is potentially mediated through epigenetic mechanisms.[78] Through modifying gene expression, epigenetic changes can thereby alter phenotypes and direct adaptation toward survival during periods of environmental stress.

Few studies to date have investigated the roles of epigenetics in AERD. In the following sections, insights from recent studies of epigenetic modifications in AERD versus other allergic asthma endotypes are discussed.

### Global Investigations of Epigenetic Modifications in Aspirin-Exacerbated Respiratory Disease

Given the dynamic regulation of expression of genes within immune and leukotriene response pathways and the corresponding lack of specific genetic markers that can explain the totality of the heterogeneity of these expression patterns, epigenetic modifications of the genome are probable contributors to AERD pathogenesis. A hallmark of epigenetic regulation is its tissue specificity, which generates specific gene expression profiles in different airway cell and tissue subsets. As discussed previously, NPs are a dominant clinical feature of AERD, are marked by eosinophilic migration and infiltration, and therefore may represent an ideal tissue model for the investigation of pathogenic cellular processes unique to AERD. A 2011 study investigated genome-wide DNA methylation levels in the context of aspirin-sensitive asthma in blood and NP samples from 5 patients with AIA and 4 patients with ATA.[79] DNA methylation profiles were interrogated using the Illumina genome-wide methylation assay chip.[79] Methylation of a total of 332 CpG sites in 296 genes was significantly increased among the patients with AIA compared with the patients with ATA, whereas 158 sites in 141 genes were significantly decreased; buffy coat DNA methylation patterns were not significantly diverse between the 2 groups.[79] Pathway analysis of the hypomethylated genes indicated enrichment in proliferation and activation of immune cells, cytokine production, and immune and inflammatory responses.[79] Alteration of these pathways through differential gene regulation may account for the spread of inflammation along the airways and proliferation of sinonasal cells leading to development of nasal polyposis. In particular, methylation patterns for 4 genes (PGDS, ALOX5AP, PTGES, and LTB4) that drive the arachidonic acid metabolism pathway that is uniquely dysregulated in AERD were altered; PGDS and ALOX5AP were hypomethylated, whereas PTGES was hypermethylated, suggesting that altered methylation patterns regulating expression of these genes could underlie aspirin hypersensitivity.[79] In addition, 2 $T_H2$ cytokine-encoding genes, IL5RA and IL10, were differentially methylated.[79] These data provide evidence that differences in gene regulation for arachidonic acid metabolism and immune response genes expressed in the upper and lower airway may account for the phenotypic differences observed between AIA and ATA.

In asthma and allergy, B lymphocytes are crucial regulators of adaptive and humoral immune responses and IgE production, which is a biomarker for hypersensitivity reactions. Furthermore, epigenetic patterns in B lymphocytes tend to be less variable across populations, which makes them a robust cellular model for comparative investigations of hypersensitivity related to allergy and asthma. Genome-wide DNA methylation profiles in $CD19^+$ B lymphocytes from a small sample of allergic asthmatics and type I hypersensitive patients were compared with profiles from patients diagnosed with AERD, bronchial asthma, and healthy controls, and the initial results were validated in an independent population.[54] DNA methylation patterns in B lymphocytes from AERD patients and healthy controls showed greater concordance than those of allergic asthmatic subjects, presumably due to the greater degree of IgE production within a specific B-cell subset in the latter group.[79]

### Functional Epigenetics of Aspirin-Exacerbated Respiratory Disease

The role of epigenetic targeting of $PGE_2$ pathway genes involved in the expansion of NPs in AERD patients was recently investigated.[80] Fibroblasts, which are the major effector cells for airway remodeling, express the arachidonic acid pathway genes that are up-regulated in AERD, and stimulation of the prostaglandin E2 receptor 2 ($EP_2$) by $PGE_2$ represses the activation and growth of these cells. Prior evidence from an epigenome-wide association study revealed that *PTGES*, the gene encoding microsomal PGE synthase-1 that converts $PGH_2$ to $PGE_2$, was hypermethylated in NP tissue from AERD subjects.[79] In addition, fibroblasts from NPs of patients with AERD have intrinsically lower expression of cyclooxygenase (COX)-2, $PGE_2$, and $EP_2$ receptor protein versus aspirin-tolerant control subjects.[81] Cahill and colleagues[80] hypothesized that an intrinsic defect in $EP_2$ expression in NP fibroblasts, potentially a result of epigenetic modification at this locus, underlies the aggressive expansion and proliferation of NPs in AERD patients. To investigate this, the investigators first isolated and cultured fibroblasts from NPs of 18 patients with AERD and 9 aspirin-tolerant patients with chronic rhinosinusitis and nasal polyposis, and nasal tissue from 8 nonasthmatic controls undergoing surgery for concha bullosa.[80] In contrast to ATA, fibroblasts from AERD patients proliferated quickly and also demonstrated persistent growth in response to treatment with $PGE_2$ as well as having reduced expression levels of the $EP_2$ receptor.[80] In addition, in AERD samples, $EP_2$ receptor mRNA was significantly up-regulated by treatment of the fibroblasts with the histone deacetylase inhibitor trichostatin A, and histone acetylation (H3K27ac) at the $EP_2$ promoter correlated strongly with baseline $EP_2$ mRNA expression levels.[80] DNA methylation at the $EP_2$ promoter in fibroblasts, however, was not significantly different, suggesting that histone modification was more likely to contribute to $EP_2$ expression in nasal fibroblasts in AERD.[80] Together, these findings support a role of epigenetic effects in AERD.

### Limitations of These Studies

There is a dearth of epigenetic investigations in AERD. A limitation of the reviewed studies is the lack of replication and poor statistical power due to small sample sizes investigated. Furthermore, to date, only a single well-designed study pursued functional characterization of specific epigenetic modifications in a cellular model of AERD. Additional epigenome-wide association studies focusing on replication, and detailed functional validation studies, are needed to clarify the extent to which specific epigenetic mechanisms contribute to AERD pathogenesis. These would be particularly informative with regard to aspirin challenge and at disease inception.

## IMPACT OF GENETICS IN THE CLINICAL MANAGEMENT OF ASPIRIN-EXACERBATED RESPIRATORY DISEASE

LTs are bioactive lipids derived from arachidonic acid (AA) that serve as immunologic mediators.[82–86] In AERD, LT overproduction has serious consequences for symptom severity and progressive airway disease.[87,88] AERD patients show significant reductions in lung function, as determined by measuring $FEV_1$, compared with non-AERD asthmatics, and significantly higher baseline and postaspirin levels of urinary $LTE_4$, the final metabolite of CysLTs, corresponding to both the severity of respiratory disease and the up-regulation of CysLTR1 expression on inflammatory cells.[89] In addition, COX-1 inhibitors (including aspirin) remove a brake on 5-LO activation, thereby increasing the baseline overproduction of LTs in AERD patients.[88] AERD patients tend to require larger doses of asthma controller medications, and treatment with LT antagonists and inhibitors (zileuton, montelukast, and zafirlukast) improves symptoms in asthma and AERD patients. These medications are routinely prescribed in higher doses to prevent or attenuate bronchospasm in AERD patients, having a positive impact on AERD treatment and improving the safety of aspirin challenges.[90] The gold standard for diagnosis of AERD is oral aspirin challenge to provoke symptomatic response.[91] During this response, CysLT production is dramatically increased, precipitating symptoms.[88,89,91,92] After diagnosis, significant improvement in asthma symptoms and slowing of NP recurrence are achieved with aspirin desensitization and daily high-dose aspirin treatment.[90] The dramatic increase in LT production immediately after aspirin challenge, and improved treatment response to montelukast in this population, provides a compelling rationale for extending investigations of LT pathway modulation in asthma to AERD. To this end, AERD represents an excellent clinical model of LT overproduction leading to a proinflammatory state to inform understanding of LT biology and treatment response.

### Pharmacogenetics

Several pharmacogenetic studies of treatment responses in AIA have been performed. Recent investigations are discussed. Due to its ability to inhibit LT-mediated airway inflammation by blocking CysLT1 receptors, montelukast treatment ideally might benefit specific asthmatic patient subgroups with overproduction of LTs as a clinical feature, including patients with aspirin hypersensitivity.[93] Montelukast as monotherapy or add-on therapy is efficient in controlling asthma and allergic rhinitis in patients with poorly controlled asthma who require corticosteroids and/or long-acting $\beta_2$-agonists.[93] Candidate gene and GWAS of anti-LT responses implicate involvement of multiple genes, including ALOX5,[32] ALOX5AP,[34,35,94–96] LTC4S,[30,34–36,87,97] CYSLTR1,[34–36,87] CYSLTR2,[34,97] ABCC1,[35,36,97–99] and OATP2B1.[100] Recently, the authors conducted the first pharmacogenomics GWAS of zileuton[101] and montelukast[102] responses in asthmatics and identified novel loci uniquely associated with both medications. Candidate gene studies of differential gene expression between non-AERD and AERD asthmatics also implicate multiple immune response and LT pathway genes, including the HLA allele DPB1,[7,74,103] CYSLTR1[7,103] and RGS7BP.[104] These findings implicate involvement of multiple genes within, and related to, the LT pathway in regulating differential responses to treatment in asthma and AERD.

A pharmacogenetic study was recently conducted with the goal of identifying prognostic factors for AERD using clinical and genetic data associated with AERD according to the clinical course of disease and response to symptom control by corticosteroids, long-acting β-agonists, and antileukotrienes.[105] A total of 122 patients with AERD were classified according to symptomatic response to aspirin rechallenge after 1 or more years of treatment with asthma controller medications; group I patients (N = 48) had negative conversions to follow-up lysine-aspirin bronchoprovocation test whereas group II patients (N = 74) showed positive responses or persistent asthma symptoms.[105] DNA samples from peripheral blood were obtained from these individuals and a case-control genetic association study of 11 candidate loci in the leukotriene and inflammatory pathways (ALOX5 1708G > 1, ALOX15 427G > A, CCR3 520T > G, CRTH2 466T > G, CYSLTR1 634C > T, IL10 1082A > G, IL13 1055C > T, LTC4S 444A > C, TGFb 509C > T, TNFa 308G > A, and HLADPB1*0301) was conducted.[105] There were no significant differences in genotype frequencies between the 2 groups, with the exception of CCR3, for which the frequency of the G allele was significantly lower in group 1 than group II.[105] A significant, genotype-dependent relationship to conversions and responses was observed, with 61% of individuals carrying CCR3 503TT showing negative conversions at follow-up and 28.6% of the patients with GT or GG genotype demonstrating negative responses, increased incidence of nasal polyposis, and a greater decline in $FEV_1$ both at baseline and after lysine-aspirin bronchoprovocation test.[105] CCR3 is a G-protein–coupled receptor that binds to several small chemoattractant proteins, known as CC-type chemokines, a class that includes the eotaxin family members that can direct eosinophils to inflammatory sites, and that are up-regulated in NP tissue.[105] These data suggest that the G allele of

*CCR3* 503 T > G is a genetic marker that can predict persistent aspirin hypersensitivity and, by virtue of its biological roles, potentially severe eosinophilia, in AERD.[105]

The role of hepatic cytochrome P450 enzymes in drug metabolism and response is well studied, and an abundance of pharmacogenetic studies has focused on the roles of these enzymes in response to various drug classes. Loss-of-function polymorphisms in *CYP2C19*, a major metabolizer of nonsteroidal anti-inflammatory drugs (NSAIDs) and AA metabolites, are more frequently expressed in Japanese patients with AERD and the percent predicted FEV $_1$ after lysine-aspirin challenge test in patents with the reference genotypes of *CYP2C19* 681G > A and 636G > A was higher than that seen in patients with GA/AA.[106] Because antileukotriene medications are more commonly prescribed for AERD, and the magnitude of treatment response to these medications among AERD patients is highly variable, discerning their routes of metabolism has relevance for therapeutic intervention, because all are either substrates and/or inhibitors of the highly polymorphic P450 enzymes. For example, montelukast is metabolized by CYP2C8,[107] zileuton is an inhibitor of CYP1A2[108] and a substrate of CYP3A4,[109] and zafirlukast is a substrate of CYP2C9.[110] Although polymorphisms that predict altered clinical pharmacokinetics of diverse drug classes have been associated with these genes, to date, no pharmacogenomic studies have investigated potential associations of these genes with variation in therapeutic responses to antileukotrienes (or other asthma medications) in AERD patients.

### Genetic Biomarkers and Predictive Tests

AERD diagnosis requires definitive confirmation by oral aspirin challenge, a time-consuming procedure during which severe clinical complications may occur. The potential of severe clinical complications arising due to provocation tests during diagnosis of AERD warrants the development of noninvasive diagnostic methods, such as biomarkers. One-fifth of severe asthmatics are unaware that they suffer from aspirin intolerance[4,111] and may, therefore, be at risk of experiencing serious exacerbations during diagnosis and otherwise. Because AERD is often underdiagnosed due to poor patient and clinical awareness of symptoms, the ability to identify novel and more precise biomarkers (genetic, epigenetic, and proteomic) associated with specific clinical features and symptoms, as well as the endotype as a whole, can assist in efforts to better identify and appropriately treat at-risk individuals. This information can be used to develop a predictive diagnostic test that can avoid complications of aspirin administration in sensitive patients, avoiding exacerbations and need for increased dosages of asthma controller medication.

Data from genetic association studies are well-suited for the development of SNP-based tests for predicting clinical phenotypes. A study conducted in 2012 sought to use existing genotype data from 109,365 SNPs genotyped in the DNA samples of 100 AERD and 100 ATA subjects from a prior GWAS to develop a prognostic SNP test for AERD.[112] A set of 8 SNPs in 8 candidate genes had sufficient discriminative power to discern AERD versus ATA.[112] In addition to GWAS data, combining gene expression and proteomic data is also useful for identifying plasma-borne biomarkers to discriminate disease phenotypes. In an effort to develop diagnostic gene and protein biomarkers of AERD using microarray data from PBMCs, Shin and colleagues[113] integrated mRNA expression profiles that were differentially expressed with regard to AERD versus ATA status with a database of secreted proteins, quantified the protein levels in plasma samples by ELISA, and assessed their discriminative ability for AERD versus ATA using ROC curve analysis. A total of 11 genes were identified as secreted proteins and validated by ELISA in patient plasma samples; among these, plasma levels of eosinophil-derived neurotoxin were significantly higher in AERD versus

ATA.[113] Furthermore, plasma eosinophil-derived neurotoxin levels showed high sensitivity and high diagnostic accuracy for predicting AERD.[113] The investigators propose that eosinophil-derived neurotoxin levels in plasma could serve as biomarker to distinguish AERD from ATA.

### Limitations of These Studies

There is tremendous clinical value in developing a noninvasive, predictive diagnostic biomarker for AERD and its clinical phenotypes using data from genetic, pharmacogenetics, and biomarker studies; however, substantial challenges must first be overcome to accomplish this goal. A major challenge for biomarker studies is the availability of robust, noise-free input data (mRNAs, SNPs, and proteins) from the ideal physiologic compartments (plasma, serum, and so forth) that can best reflect the pathologic conditions of the disease state and also be readily sampled in a clinical setting. The predictive accuracy of individual biomarkers and SNPs is highly variable and greatly depends on the modeling approach used, sample size, and phenotypic variation within the sample measured. Relevant clinical covariates and comorbidities that could affect the variation in these biomarkers, such as medication use, gender, age, tissue/cell type, and disease severity, must also be accounted for in development of accurate predictive models. Validation of the predictive models in similar data sets and clinical samples is also needed to confirm that the models can reliably and accurately predict the phenotype.

### SUMMARY

Although the molecular mechanisms that underlie AERD pathogenesis are not fully understood, genetic and epigenetic variation play a significant role. This review presents evidence from recent studies that point toward variation in diverse molecular pathways for arachidonic acid metabolism, $T_H1$ and $T_H2$ immune responses, inflammation, upper airway and nasal epithelial cell proliferation, eosinophilia, drug responses, and other pathways in AERD susceptibility and its unique clinical symptoms and response to therapy. The applications of whole-genome sequencing and next-generation technologies are anticipated to increase the likelihood of detecting potentially functional rare variants and increase the pool of associated loci. These and other association studies will require replication in diverse populations and must prioritize functional validation of new and existing associations. Epigenetic modification within B cells and NP epithelia in patients with AERD contribute an additional source of regulatory control for variation and gene expression in AERD severity. These studies are sparse, however, and also subject to the same challenges as genetic-association studies. Integration of whole-genome sequence, epigenetic, and gene expression data collected in studies with strong designs, for example, before and after ASA challenge or at disease inception, should be pursued. Finally, there is great promise in using well-validated genetic markers and proteins identified through these studies to develop predictive biomarkers that can lead to the development of noninvasive, diagnostic tests for AERD. An increased understanding of genetic and epigenetic mechanisms provides an opportunity to develop new therapeutic approaches for the diagnosis, treatment, and management of AERD.

### REFERENCES

1. Jenkins C, Costello J, Hodge L. Systematic review of prevalence of aspirin induced asthma and its implications for clinical practice. BMJ 2004;328(7437):434.
2. Vally H, Taylor ML, Thompson PJ. The prevalence of aspirin intolerant asthma (AIA) in Australian asthmatic patients. Thorax 2002;57(7):569–74.

3. Kasper L, Sladek K, Duplaga M, et al. Prevalence of asthma with aspirin hypersensitivity in the adult population of Poland. Allergy 2003;58(10):1064–6.

4. Szczeklik A, Nizankowska E, Duplaga M. Natural history of aspirin-induced asthma. AIANE Investigators. European Network on Aspirin-Induced Asthma. Eur Respir J 2000;16(3):432–6.

5. Stevenson DD. Aspirin sensitivity and desensitization for asthma and sinusitis. Curr Allergy Asthma Rep 2009;9(2):155–63.

6. Choi JH, Kim MA, Park HS. An update on the pathogenesis of the upper airways in aspirin-exacerbated respiratory disease. Curr Opin Allergy Clin Immunol 2014;14(1):1–6.

7. Palikhe NS, Kim JH, Park HS. Update on recent advances in the management of aspirin exacerbated respiratory disease. Yonsei Med J 2009;50(6):744–50.

8. Kim SH, Sanak M, Park HS. Genetics of hypersensitivity to aspirin and nonsteroidal anti-inflammatory drugs. Immunol Allergy Clin N Am 2013;33(2):177–94.

9. Busse WW, McGill KA, Horwitz RJ. Leukotriene pathway inhibitors in asthma and chronic obstructive pulmonary disease. Clin Exp Allergy 1999;29(Suppl 2): 110–5.

10. Park HS. Aspirin-sensitive asthma: recent advances in management. BioDrugs 2000;13(1):29–33.

11. Nathan RA, Kemp JP, Group AW. Efficacy of antileukotriene agents in asthma management. Ann Allergy Asthma Immunol 2001;86(6 Suppl 1):9–17.

12. Berges-Gimeno MP, Simon RA, Stevenson DD. The effect of leukotriene-modifier drugs on aspirin-induced asthma and rhinitis reactions. Clin Exp Allergy 2002; 32(10):1491–6.

13. Dahlén SE. Lipid mediator pathways in the lung: leukotrienes as a new target for the treatment of asthma. Clin Exp Allergy 1998;28(Suppl 5):141–6 [discussion: 171–3].

14. Ind PW. Anti-leukotriene intervention: is there adequate information for clinical use in asthma? Respir Med 1996;90(10):575–86.

15. Berges-Gimeno MP, Simon RA, Stevenson DD. The natural history and clinical characteristics of aspirin-exacerbated respiratory disease. Ann Allergy Asthma Immunol 2002;89(5):474–8.

16. Cowburn AS, Sladek K, Soja J, et al. Overexpression of leukotriene C4 synthase in bronchial biopsies from patients with aspirin-intolerant asthma. J Clin Invest 1998;101(4):834–46.

17. Sampson AP, Cowburn AS, Sladek K, et al. Profound overexpression of leukotriene C4 synthase in bronchial biopsies from aspirin-intolerant asthmatic patients. Int Arch Allergy Immunol 1997;113(1–3):355–7.

18. Kim SH, Choi JH, Holloway JW, et al. Leukotriene-related gene polymorphisms in patients with aspirin-intolerant urticaria and aspirin-intolerant asthma: differing contributions of ALOX5 polymorphism in Korean population. J Korean Med Sci 2005;20(6):926–31.

19. Kim SH, Bae JS, Suh CH, et al. Polymorphism of tandem repeat in promoter of 5-lipoxygenase in ASA-intolerant asthma: a positive association with airway hyperresponsiveness. Allergy 2005;60(6):760–5.

20. Sousa AR, Parikh A, Scadding G, et al. Leukotriene-receptor expression on nasal mucosal inflammatory cells in aspirin-sensitive rhinosinusitis. N Engl J Med 2002;347(19):1493–9.

21. Arm JP, O'Hickey SP, Spur BW, et al. Airway responsiveness to histamine and leukotriene E4 in subjects with aspirin-induced asthma. Am Rev Respir Dis 1989;140(1):148–53.

22. Kim SH, Oh JM, Kim YS, et al. Cysteinyl leukotriene receptor 1 promoter polymorphism is associated with aspirin-intolerant asthma in males. Clin Exp Allergy 2006;36(4):433–9.
23. Akahoshi M, Obara K, Hirota T, et al. Functional promoter polymorphism in the TBX21 gene associated with aspirin-induced asthma. Hum Genet 2005;117(1): 16–26.
24. Ying S, Meng Q, Scadding G, et al. Aspirin-sensitive rhinosinusitis is associated with reduced E-prostanoid 2 receptor expression on nasal mucosal inflammatory cells. J Allergy Clin Immunol 2006;117(2):312–8.
25. Pérez-Novo CA, Watelet JB, Claeys C, et al. Prostaglandin, leukotriene, and lipoxin balance in chronic rhinosinusitis with and without nasal polyposis. J Allergy Clin Immunol 2005;115(6):1189–96.
26. Schmid M, Göde U, Schäfer D, et al. Arachidonic acid metabolism in nasal tissue and peripheral blood cells in aspirin intolerant asthmatics. Acta Otolaryngol 1999;119(2):277–80.
27. Wang G, Zhang J, Sun H, et al. Genetic variation in members of the leukotrienes biosynthesis pathway confers risk of ischemic stroke in Eastern Han Chinese. Prostaglandins Leukot Essent Fatty Acids 2012;87(6):169–75.
28. Wang GN, Zhang JS, Cao WJ, et al. Association of ALOX5, LTA4H and LTC4S gene polymorphisms with ischemic stroke risk in a cohort of Chinese in east China. World J Emerg Med 2013;4(1):32–7.
29. Zhao N, Liu X, Wang Y, et al. Association of inflammatory gene polymorphisms with ischemic stroke in a Chinese Han population. J Neuroinflammation 2012; 9:162.
30. Lima JJ, Zhang S, Grant A, et al. Influence of leukotriene pathway polymorphisms on response to montelukast in asthma. Am J Respir Crit Care Med 2006;173(4):379–85.
31. Zhang Y, Huang H, Huang J, et al. The -444A/C polymorphism in the LTC4S gene and the risk of asthma: a meta-analysis. Arch Med Res 2012;43(6):444–50.
32. Drazen JM, Yandava CN, Dubé L, et al. Pharmacogenetic association between ALOX5 promoter genotype and the response to anti-asthma treatment. Nat Genet 1999;22(2):168–70.
33. Kim SH, Park HS. Genetic markers for differentiating aspirin-hypersensitivity. Yonsei Med J 2006;47(1):15–21.
34. Klotsman M, York TP, Pillai SG, et al. Pharmacogenetics of the 5-lipoxygenase biosynthetic pathway and variable clinical response to montelukast. Pharmacogenet Genomics 2007;17(3):189–96.
35. Lima JJ. Treatment heterogeneity in asthma: genetics of response to leukotriene modifiers. Mol Diagn Ther 2007;11(2):97–104.
36. Tantisira KG, Lima J, Sylvia J, et al. 5-lipoxygenase pharmacogenetics in asthma: overlap with Cys-leukotriene receptor antagonist loci. Pharmacogenet Genomics 2009;19(3):244–7.
37. Laidlaw TM, Boyce JA. Pathogenesis of aspirin-exacerbated respiratory disease and reactions. Immunol Allergy Clin N Am 2013;33(2):195–210.
38. Laidlaw TM, Boyce JA. Platelets in patients with aspirin-exacerbated respiratory disease. J Allergy Clin Immunol 2015;135(6):1407–14 [quiz: 1415].
39. Poon AH, Houseman EA, Ryan L, et al. Variants of asthma and chronic obstructive pulmonary disease genes and lung function decline in aging. J Gerontol A Biol Sci Med Sci 2014;69(7):907–13.
40. Allen M, Heinzmann A, Noguchi E, et al. Positional cloning of a novel gene influencing asthma from chromosome 2q14. Nat Genet 2003;35(3):258–63.

41. Kim SH, Choi H, Yoon MG, et al. Dipeptidyl-peptidase 10 as a genetic biomarker for the aspirin-exacerbated respiratory disease phenotype. Ann Allergy Asthma Immunol 2015;114(3):208–13.
42. Chang HS, Park JS, Shin HR, et al. Association analysis of FABP1 gene polymorphisms with aspirin-exacerbated respiratory disease in asthma. Exp Lung Res 2014;40(10):485–94.
43. Steinke JW, Borish L. Factors driving the aspirin exacerbated respiratory disease phenotype. Am J Rhinol Allergy 2015;29(1):35–40.
44. Kim JE, Kountakis SE. The prevalence of Samter's triad in patients undergoing functional endoscopic sinus surgery. Ear Nose Throat J 2007;86(7):396–9.
45. Robinson JL, Griest S, James KE, et al. Impact of aspirin intolerance on outcomes of sinus surgery. Laryngoscope 2007;117(5):825–30.
46. Awad OG, Lee JH, Fasano MB, et al. Sinonasal outcomes after endoscopic sinus surgery in asthmatic patients with nasal polyps: a difference between aspirin-tolerant and aspirin-induced asthma? Laryngoscope 2008;118(7): 1282–6.
47. Stevens WW, Ocampo CJ, Berdnikovs S, et al. Cytokines in Chronic Rhinosinusitis. Role in Eosinophilia and Aspirin-exacerbated Respiratory Disease. Am J Respir Crit Care Med 2015;192(6):682–94.
48. Bae JS, Pasaje CF, Park BL, et al. Genetic association analysis of CIITA variations with nasal polyp pathogenesis in asthmatic patients. Mol Med Rep 2013; 7(3):927–34.
49. Baenkler HW, Schäfer D, Hosemann W. Eicosanoids from biopsy of normal and polypous nasal mucosa. Rhinology 1996;34(3):166–70.
50. Yoshimura T, Yoshikawa M, Otori N, et al. Correlation between the prostaglandin D(2)/E(2) ratio in nasal polyps and the recalcitrant pathophysiology of chronic rhinosinusitis associated with bronchial asthma. Allergol Int 2008;57(4):429–36.
51. Adamjee J, Suh YJ, Park HS, et al. Expression of 5-lipoxygenase and cyclooxygenase pathway enzymes in nasal polyps of patients with aspirin-intolerant asthma. J Pathol 2006;209(3):392–9.
52. Benito Pescador D, Isidoro-García M, García-Solaesa V, et al. Genetic association study in nasal polyposis. J Investig Allergol Clin Immunol 2012;22(5): 331–40.
53. Batra J, Pratap Singh T, Mabalirajan U, et al. Association of inducible nitric oxide synthase with asthma severity, total serum immunoglobulin E and blood eosinophil levels. Thorax 2007;62(1):16–22.
54. Pascual M, Suzuki M, Isidoro-Garcia M, et al. Epigenetic changes in B lymphocytes associated with house dust mite allergic asthma. Epigenetics 2011;6(9): 1131–7.
55. Losol P, Kim SH, Shin YS, et al. A genetic effect of IL-5 receptor α polymorphism in patients with aspirin-exacerbated respiratory disease. Exp Mol Med 2013;45:e14.
56. Louten J, Boniface K, de Waal Malefyt R. Development and function of TH17 cells in health and disease. J Allergy Clin Immunol 2009;123(5):1004–11.
57. Kawaguchi M, Adachi M, Oda N, et al. IL-17 cytokine family. J Allergy Clin Immunol 2004;114(6):1265–73 [quiz: 1274].
58. Jung JS, Park BL, Cheong HS, et al. Association of IL-17RB gene polymorphism with asthma. Chest 2009;135(5):1173–80.
59. Park JS, Park BL, Kim MO, et al. Association of single nucleotide polymorphisms on Interleukin 17 receptor A (IL17RA) gene with aspirin hypersensitivity in asthmatics. Hum Immunol 2013;74(5):598–606.

60. Dekker JW, Nizankowska E, Schmitz-Schumann M, et al. Aspirin-induced asthma and HLA-DRB1 and HLA-DPB1 genotypes. Clin Exp Allergy 1997; 27(5):574–7.
61. Choi JH, Lee KW, Oh HB, et al. HLA association in aspirin-intolerant asthma: DPB1*0301 as a strong marker in a Korean population. J Allergy Clin Immunol 2004;113(3):562–4.
62. Park HS, Kim SH, Sampson AP, et al. The HLA-DPB1*0301 marker might predict the requirement for leukotriene receptor antagonist in patients with aspirin-intolerant asthma. J Allergy Clin Immunol 2004;114(3):688–9.
63. Esmaeilzadeh H, Nabavi M, Amirzargar AA, et al. HLA-DRB and HLA-DQ genetic variability in patients with aspirin-exacerbated respiratory disease. Am J Rhinol Allergy 2015;29(3):e63–9.
64. Steinke JW, Liu L, Huyett P, et al. Prominent role of IFN-γ in patients with aspirin-exacerbated respiratory disease. J Allergy Clin Immunol 2013;132(4): 856–65.e851-3.
65. Early SB, Barekzi E, Negri J, et al. Concordant modulation of cysteinyl leukotriene receptor expression by IL-4 and IFN-gamma on peripheral immune cells. Am J Respir Cell Mol Biol 2007;36(6):715–20.
66. Park JS, Heo JS, Chang HS, et al. Association analysis of member RAS oncogene family gene polymorphisms with aspirin intolerance in asthmatic patients. DNA Cell Biol 2014;33(3):155–61.
67. Ferro E, Goitre L, Retta SF, et al. The Interplay between ROS and Ras GTPases: Physiological and Pathological Implications. J Signal Transduct 2012;2012: 365769.
68. Takai Y, Sasaki T, Matozaki T. Small GTP-binding proteins. Physiol Rev 2001; 81(1):153–208.
69. Bertorelli G, Bocchino V, Zhuo X, et al. Heat shock protein 70 upregulation is related to HLA-DR expression in bronchial asthma. Effects of inhaled glucocorticoids. Clin Exp Allergy 1998;28(5):551–60.
70. Vignola AM, Chanez P, Polla BS, et al. Increased expression of heat shock protein 70 on airway cells in asthma and chronic bronchitis. Am J Respir Cell Mol Biol 1995;13(6):683–91.
71. Kikuchi K, Abe S, Kodaira K, et al. Heat shock protein 70 gene polymorphisms in Japanese patients with aspirin-exacerbated respiratory disease. J Investig Med 2013;61(4):708–14.
72. Milner CM, Campbell RD. Structure and expression of the three MHC-linked HSP70 genes. Immunogenetics 1990;32(4):242–51.
73. Kim SH, Cho BY, Choi H, et al. The SNP rs3128965 of HLA-DPB1 as a genetic marker of the AERD phenotype. PLoS One 2014;9(12):e111220.
74. Park BL, Kim TH, Kim JH, et al. Genome-wide association study of aspirin-exacerbated respiratory disease in a Korean population. Hum Genet 2013; 132(3):313–21.
75. Wieczfinska J, Kacprzak D, Pospiech K, et al. The whole-genome expression analysis of peripheral blood mononuclear cells from aspirin sensitive asthmatics versus aspirin tolerant patients and healthy donors after in vitro aspirin challenge. Respir Res 2015;16(1):147.
76. Shin SW, Park BL, Chang H, et al. Exonic variants associated with development of aspirin exacerbated respiratory diseases. PLoS One 2014;9(11):e111887.
77. Kim JH, Park BL, Cheong HS, et al. Genome-wide and follow-up studies identify CEP68 gene variants associated with risk of aspirin-intolerant asthma. PLoS One 2010;5(11):e13818.

78. Barker DJ. The origins of the developmental origins theory. J Intern Med 2007; 261(5):412–7.

79. Cheong HS, Park SM, Kim MO, et al. Genome-wide methylation profile of nasal polyps: relation to aspirin hypersensitivity in asthmatics. Allergy 2011;66(5): 637–44.

80. Cahill KN, Raby BA, Zhou X, et al. Impaired E Prostanoid2 Expression and Resistance to Prostaglandin E2 in Nasal Polyp Fibroblasts from Subjects with Aspirin-Exacerbated Respiratory Disease. Am J Respir Cell Mol Biol 2016; 54(1):34–40.

81. Roca-Ferrer J, Garcia-Garcia FJ, Pereda J, et al. Reduced expression of COXs and production of prostaglandin E(2) in patients with nasal polyps with or without aspirin-intolerant asthma. J Allergy Clin Immunol 2011;128(1): 66–72.e61.

82. Hammarström S. Biosynthesis and metabolism of leukotrienes. Monogr Allergy 1983;18:265–71.

83. Hammarström S. Leukotrienes. Annu Rev Biochem 1983;52:355–77.

84. Osher E, Weisinger G, Limor R, et al. The 5 lipoxygenase system in the vasculature: emerging role in health and disease. Mol Cell Endocrinol 2006;252(1–2): 201–6.

85. Salmon JA, Higgs GA. Prostaglandins and leukotrienes as inflammatory mediators. Br Med Bull 1987;43(2):285–96.

86. Sharma JN, Mohammed LA. The role of leukotrienes in the pathophysiology of inflammatory disorders: is there a case for revisiting leukotrienes as therapeutic targets? Inflammopharmacology 2006;14(1–2):10–6.

87. Duroudier NP, Tulah AS, Sayers I. Leukotriene pathway genetics and pharmacogenetics in allergy. Allergy 2009;64(6):823–39.

88. Israel E, Fischer AR, Rosenberg MA, et al. The pivotal role of 5-lipoxygenase products in the reaction of aspirin-sensitive asthmatics to aspirin. Am Rev Respir Dis 1993;148(6 Pt 1):1447–51.

89. Christie PE, Tagari P, Ford-Hutchinson AW, et al. Urinary leukotriene E4 concentrations increase after aspirin challenge in aspirin-sensitive asthmatic subjects. Am Rev Respir Dis 1991;143(5 Pt 1):1025–9.

90. Lee RU, Stevenson DD. Aspirin-exacerbated respiratory disease: evaluation and management. Allergy Asthma Immunol Res 2011;3(1):3–10.

91. McDonald JR, Mathison DA, Stevenson DD. Aspirin intolerance in asthma. Detection by oral challenge. J Allergy Clin Immunol 1972;50(4):198–207.

92. Delaney JC. The diagnosis of aspirin idiosyncrasy by analgesic challenge. Clin Allergy 1976;6(2):177–81.

93. Pacheco Y, Hosni R, Chabannes B, et al. Leukotriene B4 level in stimulated blood neutrophils and alveolar macrophages from healthy and asthmatic subjects. Effect of beta-2 agonist therapy. Eur J Clin Invest 1992;22(11):732–9.

94. Holloway JW, Barton SJ, Holgate ST, et al. The role of LTA4H and ALOX5AP polymorphism in asthma and allergy susceptibility. Allergy 2008;63(8): 1046–53.

95. Tcheurekdjian H, Via M, De Giacomo A, et al. ALOX5AP and LTA4H polymorphisms modify augmentation of bronchodilator responsiveness by leukotriene modifiers in Latinos. J Allergy Clin Immunol 2010;126(4):853–8.

96. Via M, De Giacomo A, Corvol H, et al. The role of LTA4H and ALOX5AP genes in the risk for asthma in Latinos. Clin Exp Allergy 2010;40(4):582–9.

97. Lima JJ, Blake KV, Tantisira KG, et al. Pharmacogenetics of asthma. Curr Opin Pulm Med 2009;15(1):57–62.

98. Saito S, Iida A, Sekine A, et al. Identification of 779 genetic variations in eight genes encoding members of the ATP-binding cassette, subfamily C (ABCC/MRP/CFTR. J Hum Genet 2002;47(4):147–71.

99. Weiss J, Theile D, Ketabi-Kiyanvash N, et al. Inhibition of MRP1/ABCC1, MRP2/ABCC2, and MRP3/ABCC3 by nucleoside, nucleotide, and non-nucleoside reverse transcriptase inhibitors. Drug Metab Dispos 2007;35(3):340–4.

100. Mougey EB, Feng H, Castro M, et al. Absorption of montelukast is transporter mediated: a common variant of OATP2B1 is associated with reduced plasma concentrations and poor response. Pharmacogenet Genomics 2009;19(2):129–38.

101. Dahlin A, Litonjua A, Irvin CG, et al. Genome-wide association study of leukotriene modifier response in asthma. Pharmacogenomics J 2016;16(2):151–7.

102. Dahlin A, Litonjua A, Lima JJ, et al. Genome-Wide Association Study Identifies Novel Pharmacogenomic Loci For Therapeutic Response to Montelukast in Asthma. PLoS One 2015;10(6):e0129385.

103. Shrestha Palikhe N, Kim SH, Jin HJ, et al. Genetic mechanisms in aspirin-exacerbated respiratory disease. J Allergy (Cairo) 2012;2012:794890.

104. Lee EH, Park BL, Park SM, et al. Association analysis of RGS7BP gene polymorphisms with aspirin intolerance in asthmatic patients. Ann Allergy Asthma Immunol 2011;106(4):292–300.e6.

105. Kim JH, Choi GS, Kim JE, et al. Clinical course of patients with aspirin-exacerbated respiratory disease: can we predict the prognosis? Pharmacogenomics 2014;15(4):449–57.

106. Kohyama K, Abe S, Kodaira K, et al. Arg16Gly β2-adrenergic receptor gene polymorphism in Japanese patients with aspirin-exacerbated respiratory disease. Int Arch Allergy Immunol 2011;156(4):405–11.

107. VandenBrink BM, Foti RS, Rock DA, et al. Evaluation of CYP2C8 inhibition in vitro: utility of montelukast as a selective CYP2C8 probe substrate. Drug Metab Dispos 2011;39(9):1546–54.

108. Lu P, Schrag ML, Slaughter DE, et al. Mechanism-based inhibition of human liver microsomal cytochrome P450 1A2 by zileuton, a 5-lipoxygenase inhibitor. Drug Metab Dispos 2003;31(11):1352–60.

109. Machinist JM, Mayer MD, Shet MS, et al. Identification of the human liver cytochrome P450 enzymes involved in the metabolism of zileuton (ABT-077) and its N-dehydroxylated metabolite, Abbott-66193. Drug Metab Dispos 1995;23(10):1163–74.

110. Karonen T, Laitila J, Niemi M, et al. Fluconazole but not the CYP3A4 inhibitor, itraconazole, increases zafirlukast plasma concentrations. Eur J Clin Pharmacol 2012;68(5):681–8.

111. Szczeklik A, Nizankowska E, Sanak M, et al. Aspirin-induced rhinitis and asthma. Curr Opin Allergy Clin Immunol 2001;1(1):27–33.

112. Shin SW, Park J, Kim YJ, et al. A highly sensitive and specific genetic marker to diagnose aspirin-exacerbated respiratory disease using a genome-wide association study. DNA Cell Biol 2012;31(11):1604–9.

113. Shin SW, Park JS, Park CS. Elevation of eosinophil-derived neurotoxin in plasma of the subjects with aspirin-exacerbated respiratory disease: a possible peripheral blood protein biomarker. PLoS One 2013;8(6):e66644.

# UNITED STATES POSTAL SERVICE

## Statement of Ownership, Management, and Circulation (All Periodicals Publications Except Requester Publications)

| 1. Publication Title | 2. Publication Number | 3. Filing Date |
|---|---|---|
| IMMUNOLOGY AND ALLERGY CLINICS OF NORTH AMERICA | 006 – 361 | 9/18/2016 |

| 4. Issue Frequency | 5. Number of Issues Published Annually | 6. Annual Subscription Price |
|---|---|---|
| FEB, MAY, AUG, NOV | 4 | $320.00 |

**7. Complete Mailing Address of Known Office of Publication** *(Not printer) (Street, city, county, state, and ZIP+4®)*

ELSEVIER INC.
360 PARK AVENUE SOUTH
NEW YORK, NY 10010-1710

Contact Person
STEPHEN R. BUSHING

Telephone *(Include area code)*
215-239-3688

**8. Complete Mailing Address of Headquarters or General Business Office of Publisher** *(Not printer)*

ELSEVIER INC.
360 PARK AVENUE SOUTH
NEW YORK, NY 10010-1710

**9. Full Names and Complete Mailing Addresses of Publisher, Editor, and Managing Editor** *(Do not leave blank)*

Publisher *(Name and complete mailing address)*

LINDA BELFUS, ELSEVIER INC.
1600 JOHN F KENNEDY BLVD. SUITE 1800
PHILADELPHIA, PA 19103-2899

Editor *(Name and complete mailing address)*

JESSICA MCCOOL, ELSEVIER INC.
1600 JOHN F KENNEDY BLVD. SUITE 1800
PHILADELPHIA, PA 19103-2899

Managing Editor *(Name and complete mailing address)*

ADRIANNE BRIGIDO, ELSEVIER INC.
1600 JOHN F KENNEDY BLVD. SUITE 1800
PHILADELPHIA, PA 19103-2899

**10. Owner** *(Do not leave blank. If the publication is owned by a corporation, give the name and address of the corporation immediately followed by the names and addresses of all stockholders owning or holding 1 percent or more of the total amount of stock. If not owned by a corporation, give the names and addresses of the individual owners. If owned by a partnership or other unincorporated firm, give its name and address as well as those of each individual owner. If the publication is published by a nonprofit organization, give its name and address.)*

| Full Name | Complete Mailing Address |
|---|---|
| WHOLLY OWNED SUBSIDIARY OF REED/ELSEVIER, US HOLDINGS | 1600 JOHN F KENNEDY BLVD. SUITE 1800 PHILADELPHIA, PA 19103-2899 |

**11. Known Bondholders, Mortgagees, and Other Security Holders Owning or Holding 1 Percent or More of Total Amount of Bonds, Mortgages, or Other Securities. If none, check box** ▸ ☐ None

| Full Name | Complete Mailing Address |
|---|---|
| N/A | |

**12. Tax Status** *(For completion by nonprofit organizations authorized to mail at nonprofit rates) (Check one)*
The purpose, function, and nonprofit status of this organization and the exempt status for federal income tax purposes:
☐ Has Not Changed During Preceding 12 Months
☐ Has Changed During Preceding 12 Months *(Publisher must submit explanation of change with this statement)*

| 13. Publication Title | 14. Issue Date for Circulation Data Below |
|---|---|
| IMMUNOLOGY AND ALLERGY CLINICS OF NORTH AMERICA | AUGUST 2016 |

| 15. Extent and Nature of Circulation | | | Average No. Copies Each Issue During Preceding 12 Months | No. Copies of Single Issue Published Nearest to Filing Date |
|---|---|---|---|---|
| **a. Total Number of Copies** *(Net press run)* | | | 224 | 297 |
| b. Paid Circulation *(By Mail and Outside the Mail)* | (1) | Mailed Outside-County Paid Subscriptions Stated on PS Form 3541 *(Include paid distribution above nominal rate, advertiser's proof copies, and exchange copies)* | 103 | 146 |
| | (2) | Mailed In-County Paid Subscriptions Stated on PS Form 3541 *(Include paid distribution above nominal rate, advertiser's proof copies, and exchange copies)* | 0 | 0 |
| | (3) | Paid Distribution Outside the Mails Including Sales Through Dealers and Carriers, Street Vendors, Counter Sales, and Other Paid Distribution Outside USPS® | 30 | 50 |
| | (4) | Paid Distribution by Other Classes of Mail Through the USPS *(e.g., First-Class Mail®)* | 0 | 0 |
| **c. Total Paid Distribution** *(Sum of 15b (1), (2), (3), and (4))* | | ▸ | 133 | 196 |
| d. Free or Nominal Rate Distribution *(By Mail and Outside the Mail)* | (1) | Free or Nominal Rate Outside-County Copies included on PS Form 3541 | 23 | 36 |
| | (2) | Free or Nominal Rate In-County Copies Included on PS Form 3541 | 0 | 0 |
| | (3) | Free or Nominal Rate Copies Mailed at Other Classes Through the USPS *(e.g., First-Class Mail)* | 0 | 0 |
| | (4) | Free or Nominal Rate Distribution Outside the Mail *(Carriers or other means)* | 0 | 0 |
| **e. Total Free or Nominal Rate Distribution** *(Sum of 15d (1), (2), (3) and (4))* | | ▸ | 23 | 36 |
| **f. Total Distribution** *(Sum of 15c and 15e)* | | ▸ | 156 | 232 |
| **g. Copies not Distributed** *(See Instructions to Publishers #4 (page 43))* | | ▸ | 68 | 65 |
| **h. Total** *(Sum of 15f and g)* | | ▸ | 224 | 297 |
| **i. Percent Paid** *(15c divided by 15f times 100)* | | ▸ | 85% | 84% |

* If you are claiming electronic copies, go to line 16 on page 3. If you are not claiming electronic copies, skip to line 17 on page 3.

| 16. Electronic Copy Circulation | Average No. Copies Each Issue During Preceding 12 Months | No. Copies of Single Issue Published Nearest to Filing Date |
|---|---|---|
| a. Paid Electronic Copies ▸ | 0 | 0 |
| b. Total Paid Print Copies (Line 15c) + Paid Electronic Copies (Line 16a) ▸ | 133 | 196 |
| c. Total Print Distribution (Line 15f) + Paid Electronic Copies (Line 16a) ▸ | 156 | 232 |
| d. Percent Paid (Both Print & Electronic Copies) (16b divided by 16c × 100) ▸ | 85% | 84% |

☒ I certify that 50% of all my distributed copies (electronic and print) are paid above a nominal price.

**17. Publication of Statement of Ownership**
☒ If the publication is a general publication, publication of this statement is required. Will be printed
in the NOVEMBER 2016 issue of this publication.

☐ Publication not required.

**18. Signature and Title of Editor, Publisher, Business Manager, or Owner**

STEPHEN R. BUSHING - INVENTORY DISTRIBUTION CONTROL MANAGER

Date 9/18/2016

I certify that all information furnished on this form is true and complete. I understand that anyone who furnishes false or misleading information on this form or who omits material or information requested on the form may be subject to criminal sanctions (including fines and imprisonment) and/or civil sanctions (including civil penalties).

PS Form **3526**, July 2014 *(Page 3 of 4)* PRIVACY NOTICE: See our privacy policy on www.usps.com.

PS Form 3526, July 2014 *(Page 1 of 4 (see instructions page 4))* PSN 7530-01-000-9931 PRIVACY NOTICE: See our privacy policy on www.usps.com.

Printed and bound by CPI Group (UK) Ltd, Croydon, CR0 4YY

07/10/2024

01040506-0012